Dieter E. Pongratz, Prof. Dr. med.
Siegfried Mense, Prof. Dr. med.
Michael Spaeth, Dr. med. MD
Editors

Soft Tissue Pain Syndromes: Clinical Diagnosis and Pathogenesis

Soft Tissue Pain Syndromes: Clinical Diagnosis and Pathogenesis has been co-published simultaneously as *Journal of Musculoskeletal Pain*, Volume 12, Numbers 3/4 2004.

Pre-publication
REVIEWS,
COMMENTARIES,
EVALUATIONS . . .

"INVALUABLE to every doctor, therapist, resident, teacher, researcher, administrator, and practitioner. . . . ESSENTIAL READING for all medical practitioners in this field. . . . Provides a unique overview of current knowledge and future trends in managing pain syndromes. Impressive in its scholarship, this book brings together leading experts from around the world in the field of soft tissue pain syndromes."

Frankie L. Burget, OTR, RMT/MI, CNDT, CWE, FACW
Licensed Therapist
Windsong Therapy and Wellness, Inc.
Bedford, Texas

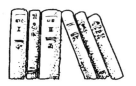

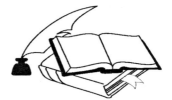

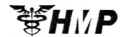

The Haworth Medical Press®
An Imprint of The Haworth Press, Inc.

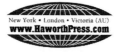

New York • London • Victoria (AU)
www.HaworthPress.com

Soft Tissue Pain Syndromes:
Clinical Diagnosis
and Pathogenesis

Soft Tissue Pain Syndromes: Clinical Diagnosis and Pathogenesis has been co-published simultaneously as *Journal of Musculoskeletal Pain*, Volume 12, Numbers 3/4 2004.

Soft Tissue Pain Syndromes: Clinical Diagnosis and Pathogenesis, edited by Dieter E. Pongratz, Prof. Dr. med., Siegfried Mense, Prof. Dr. med., and Michael Spaeth, Dr. med. MD (Vol. 12, No. 3/4, 2004). *Selections from the 2004 International MYOPAIN Society's Sixth World Congress held in Munich, Germany, examining of the state-of-the-art in pain mechanisms, myofascial pain syndrome, fibromyalgia syndrome, and inflammatory myopathies.*

International MYOPAIN Society–MYOPAIN 2004: Abstracts from the Sixth World Congress on Myofascial Pain and Fibromyalgia, Munich, Germany, July 18-July 22, 2004 (Vol. 12, Suppl. #9, 2004). *Experts examine recent developments in the fields of myofascial pain and fibromyalgia.*

The Fibromyalgia Syndrome: A Clinical Case Definition for Practitioners, edited by I. Jon Russell, MD, PhD (Vol. 11, No. 4, 2003). *Establishes an expert consensus toward a working case definition of fibromyalgia syndrome and a working guide to its management for physicians in Canada.*

The Clinical Neurobiology of Fibromyalgia and Myofascial Pain: Therapeutic Implications, edited by Robert M. Bennett, MD (Vol. 10, No. 1/2, 2002). *Covers the latest developments in pain research: examines the results of a wide scope of basic and applied research on soft-tissue pain.*

International MYOPAIN Society–MYOPAIN '01: Abstracts from the 5th World Congress on Myofascial Pain and Fibromyalgia, Portland, Oregon, USA, September 9-September 13, 2001 (Vol. 9, Suppl. #5, 2001)

Muscle Pain, Myofascial Pain, and Fibromyalgia: Recent Advances, edited by Leonardo Vecchiet, MD, and Maria Adele Giamberardino, MD (Vol. 7, No. 1/2, 1999). *Covers the latest developments in musculoskeletal pain that were presented at the MYOPAIN '98 Congress in Silvi Marina, Italy.*

MYOPAIN '98: Abstracts from the 4th World Congress on Myofascial Pain and Fibromyalgia, Silvi Marina [TE], ITALY, August 24-August 27, 1998, edited by Leonardo Vecchiet, MD, and Maria Adele Giamberardino, MD (Vol. 6, Suppl. #2, 1998).

The Neuroscience and Endocrinology of Fibromyalgia, edited by Stanley R. Pillemer, MD (Vol. 6, No. 3, 1998). *"I recommend this book to all health care providers who want to offer the most up-to-date therapy for their patients with fibromyalgia." [David Borestein, MD, Clinical Professor of Medicine, The George Washington University Medical Center, Arthritis and Rheumatism]*

Muscle Pain Syndromes and Fibromyalgia: Pressure Algometry for Quantification of Diagnosis and Treatment Outcome, edited by Andrew A. Fischer, MD, PhD (Vol. 6, No. 1, 1998). *"Should help researchers in developing new and expanded studies for the appropriate role of pressure algometry." [Martin Grabois, MD, Professor and Chairman, Physical Medicine and Rehabilitation, Baylor College of Medicine, Houston, Texas]*

Musculoskeletal Pain Emanating from the Head and Neck: Current Concepts in Diagnosis, Management, and Cost Containment, edited by Murray E. Allen, MD (Vol. 4, No. 4, 1996). *"Exciting because it contains a distillation of recent research that is of value to all who treat and serve those with whiplash-related injuries." [National Association of Rehabilitation Professionals in the Private Sector]*

Clinical Overview and Pathogenesis of the Fibromyalgia Syndrome, Myofascial Pain Syndrome, and Other Pain Syndromes, edited by I. Jon Russell, MD, PhD (Vol. 4, No. 1/2, 1996). *The featured speakers at the MYOPAIN '95 Third World Congress are here distilled into an anthology that represents a state of the art in fibromyalgia syndrome and myofascial pain syndrome from that conference.*

MYOPAIN '95: Abstracts from the 3rd World Congress on Myofascial Pain and Fibromyalgia, San Antonio, Texas, USA, July 30-August 3, 1995, edited by I. Jon Russell, MD, PhD (Vol. 3, Suppl. #1, 1995). *An excellent resource that allows physicians, dentists, researchers, and others working in this field to access key information as presented by specialists worldwide who work with and research chronic muscle pain.*

Fibromyalgia, Chronic Fatigue Syndrome, and Repetitive Strain Injury: Current Concepts in Diagnosis, Management, Disability, and Health Economics, edited by Andrew Chalmers, MD, Geoffrey Owen Littlejohn, MD, Irving Salit, MD, and Frederick Wolfe, MD (Vol. 3, No. 2, 1995). *"The information and original research presented is relevant and useful for understanding some of the global research being conducted on these disorders. . . . It would be most useful as an addition to a scientific/medical library." [Annals of Pharmacotherapy]*

The Fibromyalgia Syndrome: Current Research and Future Directions in Epidemiology, Pathogenesis, and Treatment, edited by Stanley R. Pillemer, MD (Vol. 2, No. 3, 1994). *"This highly informative and well-referenced text is recommended to both students and practitioners." [Annals of Pharmacotherapy]*

Musculoskeletal Pain, Myofascial Pain Syndrome, and the Fibromyalgia Syndrome: Proceedings from the Second World Congress on Myofascial Pain and Fibromyalgia, edited by Søren Jacobsen, MD, Bente Danneskiold-Samsøe, MD, PhD, and Birger Lund, MD, PhD (Vol. 1, No. 3/4, 1993). *"Packed with state-of-the-art information. . . . An important contribution to our understanding of myofascial pain syndrome, fibromyalgia, and musculoskeletal pain, and will be useful to both patients and health care providers." [Lifeline [National Chronic Pain Outreach Association]]*

Soft Tissue Pain Syndromes:
Clinical Diagnosis
and Pathogenesis

Dieter E. Pongratz, Prof. Dr. med.
Siegfried Mense, Prof. Dr. med.
Michael Spaeth, Dr. med. MD
Editors

Soft Tissue Pain Syndromes: Clinical Diagnosis and Pathogenesis has been co-published simultaneously as *Journal of Musculoskeletal Pain*, Volume 12, Numbers 3/4 2004.

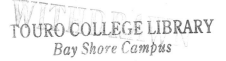
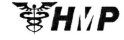

The Haworth Medical Press®
An Imprint of The Haworth Press, Inc.

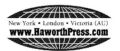

New York • London • Victoria (AU)
www.HaworthPress.com

BS

Published by

The Haworth Medical Press®, 10 Alice Street, Binghamton, NY 13904-1580 USA

The Haworth Medical Press® is an imprint of The Haworth Press, Inc., 10 Alice Street, Binghamton, NY 13904-1580 USA.

Soft Tissue Pain Syndromes: Clinical Diagnosis and Pathogenesis has been co-published simultaneously as *Journal of Musculoskeletal Pain*, Volume 12, Numbers 3/4 2004.

The development, preparation, and publication of this work has been undertaken with great care. However, the publisher, employees, editors, and agents of The Haworth Press and all imprints of The Haworth Press, Inc., including The Haworth Medical Press® and Pharmaceutical Products Press®, are not responsible for any errors contained herein or for consequences that may ensue from use of materials or information contained in this work. Opinions expressed by the author(s) are not necessarily those of The Haworth Press, Inc. With regard to case studies, identities and circumstances of individuals discussed herein have been changed to protect confidentiality. Any resemblance to actual persons, living or dead, is entirely coincidental.

Cover design by Katie R. Johnson.

Library of Congress Cataloging-in-Publication Data

World Congress on Myofascial Pain and Fibromyalgia (6th : 2004 : Munich, Germany)
Soft tissue pain syndromes : clinical diagnosis and pathogenesis / Dieter E. Pongratz, Siegfried Mense, Michael Spaeth, editors.
p. ; cm.
"Co-published simultaneously as Journal of musculoskeletal pain, volume 12, numbers 3/4 2004."
Includes bibliographical references and index.
ISBN-13: 978-0-7890-3138-9 (soft cover : alk. paper)
ISBN-10: 0-7890-3138-8 (soft cover : alk. paper)
1. Soft tissue injuries–Congresses. 2. Pain–Congresses. 3. Fibromyalgia–Congresses. I. Pongratz, Dieter E. (Dieter Erich) II. Mense, Siegfried. III. Spaeth, Michael. IV. Title.
[DNLM: 1. Myofascial Pain Syndromes–Congresses. 2. Fibromyalgia–Congresses. 3. Low Back Pain–Congresses. W1 JO775RK v.12 no.3/4 / WE 550 W927s 2006]
RC925.5.S64 2006
616.7'42–dc22
2005022174

3/26/07

Indexing, Abstracting & Website/Internet Coverage

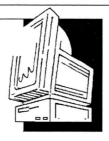

This section provides you with a list of major indexing & abstracting services and other tools for bibliographic access. That is to say, each service began covering this periodical during the year noted in the right column. Most Websites which are listed below have indicated that they will either post, disseminate, compile, archive, cite, or alert their own Website users with research-based content from this work. [This list is as current as the copyright date of this publication.]

Abstracting, Website/Indexing Coverage ....Year When Coverage Began

- *AnalgesiaFile, Dannemiller Memorial Educational Foundation, Texas*
  <http://www.pain.com>.. 2003

- *Behavioral Medicine Abstracts [Annals of Behavioral Medicine]* 1994

- *Behavioral Medicine Abstracts [Pain Evaluation and Treatment Institute]*.............. 1997

- *Biology Digest [in print & online] <http://www.infotoday.com>*....................... 2000

- *Cambridge Scientific Abstracts [Calcium & Calcified Tissue Abstracts/Health & Safety*
  Science Abstracts] <http://www.csa.com> 1993

- *Centre Regional D'Exploration des Myalgies <http://www.infomyalgie.com>* 1996

- *CFS-NEWS* 1999

- *CINAHL [Cumulative Index to Nursing & Allied Health Literature], in print, EBSCO,*
  and SilverPlatter, DataStar, and PaperChase. [Support materials include Subject
  Heading List, Database Search Guide, and instructional video]
  <http://www.cinahl.com> 1996

- *Current Contents/Clinical Medicine <http://www.isinet.com>* 1997

- *e-psyche, LLC <http://www.e-psyche.net>*.. 2001

- *EBSCOhost Electronic Journals Service [EJS] <http://ejournals.ebsco.com>* 2001

- *EMBASE.com [The Power of EMBASE + MEDLINE Combined]*
  <http://www.embase.com> 1993

- *EMBASE/Excertpa Medica Secondary Publishing Division. Included in newsletters,*
  review journals, major reference works, magazines & abstract journals.
  <http://www.elsevier.nl>.. 1993

- *Environmental Sciences and Pollution Management [Cambridge Scientific Abstracts*
  Internet Database Service] <http://www.csa.com> 1993

- *Excerpta Medica . . . See EMBASE/Excerpta Medica*............................... 1993

[continued]

Special Bibliographic Notes related to special journal issues
[separates] and indexing/abstracting:

- indexing/abstracting services in this list will also cover material in any "separate" that is co-published simultaneously with Haworth's special thematic journal issue or DocuSerial. Indexing/abstracting usually covers material at the article/chapter level.
- monographic co-editions are intended for either non-subscribers or libraries which intend to purchase a second copy for their circulating collections.
- monographic co-editions are reported to all jobbers/wholesalers/approval plans. The source journal is listed as the "series" to assist the prevention of duplicate purchasing in the same manner utilized for books-in-series.
- to facilitate user/access services all indexing/abstracting services are encouraged to utilize the co-indexing entry note indicated at the bottom of the first page of each article/chapter/contribution.
- this is intended to assist a library user of any reference tool [whether print, electronic, online, or CD-ROM] to locate the monographic version if the library has purchased this version but not a subscription to the source journal.
- individual articles/chapters in any Haworth publication are also available through the Haworth Document Delivery Service [HDDS].

Soft Tissue Pain Syndromes: Clinical Diagnosis and Pathogenesis

CONTENTS

Preface   xiii
I. Jon Russell

PRESIDENT'S ADDRESS

Three Years Later: Presidential Address to MYOPAIN '04   1
Robert M. Bennett

MYOFASCIAL PAIN SYNDROME

Mechanisms of the Transition from Acute to Chronic Pain   13
Walter Zieglgänsberger

New Aspects of Myofascial Trigger Points: Etiological and Clinical   15
David G. Simons

Differential Diagnosis of Trigger Points   23
Robert Gerwin

Trigger Points as a Cause of Orofacial Pain   29
Sandro Palla

Myofascial Pain Therapy   37
Chang-Zern Hong

FIBROMYALGIA PAIN SYNDROME

Pain and the Neuroendocrine System   45
Gunther Neeck

Developments in the Fibromyalgia Syndrome   47
I. Jon Russell

Diagnostic Criteria and Differential Diagnosis of the Fibromyalgia Syndrome   59
Robert M. Bennett

Fibromyalgia: Novel Therapeutic Aspects   65
Carol S. Burckhardt

Fibromyalgia: Novel Drug Therapies   73
Leslie Crofford

PAINFUL MYOPATHIES AND "IDIOPATHIC" LOW BACK PAIN

Painful Myopathies–Metabolism of Muscle Cells and Metabolic Myopathies   75
    Heinz Reichmann
    Jochen Schaefer

Clinical Presentation and Therapy of Idiopathic Inflammatory Myopathies   85
    Frederick W. Miller

Idiopathic Low Back Pain: Classification and Differential Diagnosis   93
    Bente Danneskiold-Samsøe
    Else Marie Bartels

Central Nervous Sequelae of Local Muscle Pain   101
    Siegfried Mense
    U. Hoheisel

Therapy for Idiopathic Low Back Pain   111
    H. Bliddal

INAUGURAL INCOMING PRESIDENT'S ADDRESS

Scientific Aspects and Clinical Signs of Muscle Pain   121
    Dieter E. Pongratz
    Matthias Vorgerd
    Benedikt G. H. Schoser

Index   129

ABOUT THE EDITORS

Dieter E. Pongratz, Prof. Dr. med., is Professor of Neurology and Internal Medicine at the University of Munich. Since 1980, he has been the leader of the Friedrich-Baur-Institute there. He is an educator, clinical investigator, and physician caring for patients with neuromuscular diseases. His research interests have focused on the clinical aspects and myopathological findings in patients with neuromuscular diseases. This work has resulted in the publication of about 300 original papers and the editing of books covering topics like clinical neurology, muscle disease, and differential diagnosis in internal medicine. He is a member of many professional societies and is currently President of the International MYOPAIN Society.

Siegfried Mense, Prof. Dr. med., is Professor of Anatomy and Cell Biology at Heidelberg University. He has a university education in both physiology and anatomy, and for more than 30 years he has studied the neuroanatomy and neurophysiology of muscle pain in animal experiments. Recently, the main focus of his research activities has been mechanisms of the transition from acute to chronic muscle pain. In addition to a large number of publications in highly ranking journals, he published–together with David G. Simons and I. Jon Russell–a book on basic and clinical aspects of muscle pain in 2001. One of his goals in research and continuing education is to bridge the unnecessarily wide gap between basic and clinical research. He has been a member of the council of the German chapter of the IASP for more than 10 years, and is currently Chairman of the German Pain Foundation.

Michael Spaeth, Dr. med. MD, is an internist and rheumatologist and a member of many professional societies. Since 1992, he has been a physician and clinical investigator at the University of Munich [Friedrich-Baur-Institute]. His research interests have focused on Sjögren's syndrome, immunogenic myopathies, and fibromyalgia syndrome. He has published both original articles and book chapters. He has been the main investigator of several clinical trials in fibromyalgia and has been caring for patients with all conditions presenting with muscle pain. In 2003, he became the Senior Physician for rheumatology at the Friedrich-Baur-Institute. He is now the co-leader of a new outpatient department caring for patients with rheumatic diseases and fibromyalgia and is performing clinical trials.

Preface

The International MYOPAIN Society's Sixth World Congress, MYOPAIN 2004, was held in the "Gem of Bavaria," Munich, Germany from July 18-22, 2004. The four main topics of this MYOPAIN meeting were the myofascial pain syndrome, the fibromyalgia syndrome, painful myopathies, and low back pain.

While the cultural flavor of each MYOPAIN meeting has been unique to its host country, the clinical and scientific objectives have always been the same–to present the most up-to-date concepts derived from basic and applied research regarding soft-tissue pain conditions, to facilitate communication between clinicians and investigators, and to gain renewed momentum for three more years of productivity.

The local co-hosts of MYOPAIN 2004 were Prof. Dr. med. Dieter Pongratz of Munich, Germany, and Prof. Dr. med. Siegfried Mense of Heidelberg, Germany. They and their committee [Robert M. Bennett, MD, USA; Leslie Crofford, MD, USA; Salvatore DiMauro, MD, PhD, USA; Chang-Zern Hong, MD, Taiwan; Frederick W. Miller, MD, PhD, USA; I. Jon Russell, MD, PhD, USA; and Dave Simons, MD, DSc [Hon], USA] organized the scientific program for the Congress. Dr. Michael Spaeth of Munich was the local arrangements coordinator. In recognition of their outstanding contributions to a successful MYOPAIN meeting, the Professors Drs. med. Pongratz and Mense and Dr. med. Spaeth, MD, are also recognized as the honorary editors of this publication.

The local arrangements coordinator for MYOPAIN 2004 provided the meeting attendees and guests with a grand tour of Munich and its environs. In addition, there was a special catered evening at Munich's incredible Neue Pinakothek Museum of Fine Art. The meeting really had an international flavor with attendees from 38 countries.

The scientific program offered a balanced view of the soft tissue pain syndromes from basic science to clinical management. In a previously published *Journal of Musculoskeletal Pain* supplement, you will find over 150 original abstracts that were accepted for presentation at the meeting. This publication offers a synopsis of the plenary presentations at MYOPAIN 2004.

The Continuing Medical Education surveys and unsolicited comments regarding the meeting clearly indicated that the MYOPAIN 2004 meeting was a resounding success.

The IMS is growing in strength and influence on the world stage as its single-minded focus on soft tissue pain becomes more widely recognized. There is much more yet to be done. If you are not yet a member of the IMS, but are interested in expanding knowledge about soft tissue pain disorders and in improving medical care for people experiencing soft tissue pain, IMS needs you. Your ideas, your vision, your ability, and your energy are needed to help lead IMS into the future. Your membership and your commitment will make the difference!

The Seventh World Congress, MYOPAIN 2007, will be held in Washington, DC, August 19 to 23, 2007. We hope to see your there.

I. Jon Russell, MD, PhD

[Haworth co-indexing entry note]: "Preface" Russell, I. Jon. Co-published simultaneously in *Journal of Musculoskeletal Pain* [The Haworth Medical Press, an imprint of The Haworth Press, Inc.] Vol. 12, No. 3/4, 2004, p. xvii: and: *Soft Tissue Pain Syndromes: Clinical Diagnosis and Pathogenesis* [ed: Dieter E. Pongratz, Siegfried Mense, and Michael Spaeth] The Haworth Medical Press, an imprint of The Haworth Press, Inc., 2004, p. xiii. Single or multiple copies of this article are available for a fee from The Haworth Document Delivery Service [1-800-HAWORTH, 9:00 a.m. - 5:00 p.m. [EST]. E-mail address: docdelivery@haworthpress.com].

Three Years Later:
Presidential Address to MYOPAIN '04

Robert M. Bennett

The last MYOPAIN Congress was held in Portland, Oregon from September 9 to September 12, 2001. For those present, this meeting will forever be defined by the tragic events that occurred on the east coast of the United States on the morning of September 11. The membership observed a minute of silence and determined to continue with the meeting, despite the powerful emotions and uncertainties that surrounded those few days. Since that day the world has, in many ways, become a less secure place with further terrorist attacks, new wars, and realigned political alliances. However, scientific research into the disorders that form a common basis for the International MYOPAIN Society has continued unabated. In the interval between 2001 and June of 2004 there were 815 fibromyalgia syndrome [FMS] articles and 185 myofascial pain articles referenced in the National Library of Medicine database [selected under the title and/or abstract]. There were, of course, many additional articles on these subjects that were published in the *Journal of Musculoskeletal Pain*. In this short review I will highlight those articles I found to be of particular interest or relevance.

WORLD TRADE CENTER DISASTER AND PSYCHOLOGICAL DISTRESS

Psychological stressors, particularly those that are persistent, are well recognized by clinicians as apparent triggering factors in the initiation of FMS. Many FMS patients report that stressful situations exacerbate their pain (1). Despite this well recognized clinical association there had been few formal studies of stressors and FMS until the relatively new entity of post-traumatic stress disorder [PTSD] became well recognized. One of the most common psychiatric complications of war is PTSD (2). In this disorder it is thought that psychological reactions to remembrances of past traumatic events trigger bodily changes. Over the last few years there have been several studies documenting an association of FMS with PTSD (35).

Robert M. Bennett, MD, FRCP, is Professor of Medicine, Oregon Health and Science University, Portland, OR 97201 USA.

[Haworth co-indexing entry note]: "Three Years Later: Presidential Address to MYOPAIN '04." Bennett, Robert M. Co-published simultaneously in *Journal of Musculoskeletal Pain* [The Haworth Medical Press, an imprint of The Haworth Press, Inc.] Vol. 12, No. 3/4, 2004, pp. 1-12; and: *Soft Tissue Pain Syndromes: Clinical Diagnosis and Pathogenesis* [ed: Dieter E. Pongratz, Siegfried Mense, and Michael Spaeth] The Haworth Medical Press, an imprint of The Haworth Press, Inc., 2004, pp. 1-12. Single or multiple copies of this article are available for a fee from The Haworth Document Delivery Service [1-800-HAWORTH. 9:00 a.m. - 5:00 p.m. [EST]. E-mail address: docdelivery@haworthpress.com].

As severe stressors have often been linked to the onset of FMS symptomatology, it was of interest to determine whether the events of September 11, 2001 [9/11] had an impact on the prevalence or severity of FMS. Two such studies have been reported on the same group of patients. In the first study advantage was taken of the fact that 1,312 women living in the New York/New Jersey metropolitan area had been surveyed for pain and psychological distress just prior to 9/11. These same subjects were reassessed by questionnaire six months following 9/11. It was found that symptoms of widespread pain did not increase significantly following 9/11. Furthermore, close exposure to the World Trade Center and depressive symptomatology prior to 9/11 were not correlated with new onset FMS like symptoms. It was concluded that major stressors and depressive symptoms are unlikely to be of major importance in the pathogenesis of FMS (6). In a separate analysis of these same patients a questionnaire regarding PTSD symptoms was added. It was found that the probability of having PTSD symptoms was three times greater in women with FMS like symptoms as assessed either pre- or post 9/11. It was concluded that FMS and PTSD may share common biological risk factors (7).

A particularly interesting report involved eight FMS patients living in the Washington DC area whose pain was being monitored with a handheld computer–as part of a drug study. The monitoring extended over a period from August 28 to September 25, 2001 and did not show any significant increase in pain post 9/11 (8).

There have been many psychological studies following events of 9/11 and many have shown an association with subsequent psychological problems (9-12). For instance, subjects who were directly exposed to a disaster and repeatedly watched television images of people falling or jumping from the towers of the World Trade Center were more likely to have depressive symptoms and PTSD (13). I suspect that the six month follow-up studies of FMS related symptoms maybe too short a time to fully assess the effects of the 9/11 experience on the subsequent development of FMS.

The psychobiological mechanism whereby mental stress can lead to bodily symptoms is a very active area of research in disorders as diverse as coronary artery disease, altered immunity, and FMS. A common denominator in these disorders is an elevation of the inflammatory cytokines (14). There is evidence that chronic stress can eventually lead to an impaired stress response, as originally envisaged by Selye and there is some evidence for such an impaired hypothalamic pituitary adrenal [HPA] axis response to stressors in FMS patients (15) as well as PTSD (16). Pro-inflammatory cytokines activate the HPA axis which in turn attempts to modulate inflammatory response. It is been hypothesized that an impaired cortisol response to stressors may in part be responsible for elevated levels of pro-inflammatory cytokines that have been reported in situations of chronic stress (17). Another central pathway that may be involved in the development of stress-induced hyperalgesia is the ventral tegmental-mesolimbic dopamine system which projects to the nucleus accumbens (18). Acute stressors have an analgesic effect via a release of endogenous opioids and substance P within the ventral tegmental region with subsequent stimulation of dopamine output by the nucleus accumbens (19). On the other hand, prolonged unavoidable stress down regulates dopamine secretion by the nucleus accumbens and results in hyperalgesia. It has been hypothesized that a stress-related reduction of dopaminergic tone within the nucleus accumbens contributes to the development of hyperalgesia in the context of chronic stress and thus plays a role in the pathogenesis of FMS (20).

EPIDEMIOLOGICAL STUDIES

Two population epidemiological studies, one from Brazil (21) and the other from Spain (22) reported FMS prevalence at 2.5 percent and 2.4 percent respectively. In the Brazil study, FMS was the second most common [35 percent] condition seen by rheumatologists.

Critics of the FMS concept often resort to the argument that providing patients with a diagnostic label is detrimental as it "enables people experiencing the usual aches and pains of human existence to legitimize dysfunctional behaviors." This notion was directly tested by the London Fibromyalgia Epidemiology Study Group (23). Seventy-two subjects with newly labeled FMS [identified by a postal screening of 3,395 noninstitutionalized adults] were entered into the study and prediagnosis FMS symptomatology Fibromyalgia Impact Questionnaire, healthcare utilization, and reported work disability were assessed at 18 and 36 month follow-ups. There was a statistically significant improvement in the newly diagnosed cases with respect to number of symptoms, severity of major symptoms, and satisfaction with health. No other differences in clinical status or health service utilization occurred. It is concluded that diagnosing a patient with FMS does not have the adverse effect that has been postulated by some critics.

In another carefully designed study the London Fibromyalgia Group examined the question as to whether FMS symptomatology is driven by litigation or compensation availability (24). This epidemiological study was conducted on 242 Amish adults, a segregated population living a simple life without resource to litigation and/or compensation issues. The prevalence of FMS was 10.4 percent in women and 3.7 percent in men. This is one of the highest FMS prevalence rates that have been found in population studies, and strongly argues against the concept that FMS symptomatology is driven by secondary gain.

Fibromyalgia is generally considered to be a very troublesome disorder that seriously impacts quality of life but has no impact on life expectancy. This assumption was challenged by an epidemiological study from northeast England on 6,565 subjects with widespread body pain who participated in health surveys conducted in 1991 and 1992 (25). In 1991, 15 percent of subjects were classified as having widespread pain and 48 percent as having regional pain. At follow-up in 1992, 365 subjects had developed malignancies. Having widespread pain gave an overall relative risk for malignancy of 1.61 and having regional pain a relative risk of 1.19. Widespread pain was most strongly correlated with breast cancer [RR 3.67], prostate [RR 3.46], large bowel [RR 2.35], and lung cancer [RR 2.04]. Patients reporting widespread pain had an increased risk of death [MRR 1.82].

CENTRAL SENSITIZATION

The last three years have provided unequivocal evidence that a major component of pain experience in FMS is related to central amplification of sensory impulses–i.e., "central sensitization." A summary of this evidence is provided in Table 1.

In this respect one important component for a biological basis for FMS symptomatology has been demonstrated. Although the increased understanding of this phenomenon may ex-

TABLE 1

Experimental finding	Reference[s]
Elevated CSF levels of substance P	(26-28)
Elevated CSF levels of dynorphin	(29)
Elevated CSF levels of nerve growth factor	(30)
Enhanced temporal summation of cutaneous thermal sensation	(31)
Enhanced temporal summation of muscle pressure sensation	(32)
Enhanced somatosensory potentials in response to skin stimulation	(33;34)
Magnified response to intramuscular injections of hypertonic saline	(35)
A lower threshold for elicitation of the nociceptive flexion reflex	(36;37)
Pain reduction after infusion of ketamine [an NMDA receptor antagonist]	(38;39)
Elevated plasma levels of neuropeptides Y	(40)
Impaired activation of descending inhibitory pathways	(41;42)
Increased activity of cerebral pain processing areas on fMRI	(43;44)
Decreased thalamic activity on functional brain scans	(45;46)

CSF = Cerebral spinal fluid; NMDA = N-methyl-D-aspartate; fMRI = functional magnetic resonance imaging

plain many of the somatic symptoms of FMS patients, it probably will not explain symptoms related to fatigue, autonomic dysfunction, cognitive deficits, and sleep disturbance. However, I hope that the elucidation of at least one part of the FMS puzzle will deter prospective authors from starting their papers with "the cause of FMS is unknown"!

PERIPHERAL PAIN GENERATORS

While central sensitization is now generally accepted as a major component of nociceptive amplification in FMS, the cause of central sensitization is still a matter of some conjecture (47). Peripheral pain generators provide the most obvious link with central sensitization. There is an impressive body of evidence both from animal experiments and the human experience that persistent nociceptive input leads to temporal summation [i.e., wind-up], with a potential to cause long-lasting changes within the central nervous system [neuroplasticity] that can result in a chronic pain state. In this respect nociceptive impulses from muscle are especially potent at effecting wind-up (48) and recent studies have indicated that repetitive stimulation of muscle in FMS patients induces more pronounced wind-up than repetitive thermal stimulation of skin (32). Maybe the "old fashioned" concept that muscle abnormalities play a central role in the pathogenesis of FMS will again become popular! Nearly all FMS patients report that their pain is muscular in origin and aggravated by overexertion. Physicians who recognize focal muscle pain generators in FMS and treat with injection therapy are especially aware that myofascial trigger points are a sine qua non of the FMS experience. Thus an improved understanding of the biological basis of myofascial trigger points and their role in the generation of central sensitization will be an important area in ongoing research endeavors. The old term of "fibrositis" (49) was abandoned in 1990 because there was no evidence of inflammation in the connective tissue between muscle bundles. Subsequent studies failed to reveal any specific abnormality in the muscles of FMS patients compared to healthy individuals. However, abnormalities are found in the muscles of FMS patients, but they are not spe-

cific or uniform (50). More recently several P-31 magnetic resonance spectroscopy studies have reported an increased prevalence of phosphodiester peaks [PDE] in FMS muscle compared to healthy individuals (51-56). An increased occurrence of PDE peaks results from damage to sarcolemmal membranes from a variety of insults (57-59). The cause of these insults in FMS patients is thought to be exercise-induced muscle damage (60,61). If this notion is correct a logical corollary is that subjects destined to develop FMS have a predisposition for developing myofascial trigger points. Possible causes of this predisposition would include the sarcopenia of normal aging (62), reduced anabolism [as occurs in hypothyroidism, growth hormone deficiency, and low testosterone levels], and progressive deconditioning as a result of an unhealthy lifestyle. Another intriguing possibility, that has yet to be explored in FMS, is increased rates of the deleterious mitochondrial deoxyribonucleic acid [DNA] mutations (63-65). In this respect a recent study of FMS patients reporting increased DNA fragmentation and abnormalities in mitochondria number and structure is of great interest (66).

CYTOKINES

Elevated levels of pro-inflammatory cytokines have been implicated in the hyperalgesia and fatigue of flu-like illnesses (67). Thus speculation has arisen as to whether cytokines may play a role in the central sensitization of FMS subjects, as there is a well described association of FMS with potent stimuli for a pro-inflammatory cytokine response such as hepatitis C (68) and treatment of malignancies with interferon-alpha or interleukin-2 (69).

The muscle aches and fatigue that commonly accompany viral illnesses such as influenza are referred to as "the sickness response" (70). It is thought that this response is mediated mainly by pro-inflammatory cytokines and activation of glial cells (71).

Two recent papers that have reported increased serum levels of interleukin [IL] 8 [but normal serum levels of IL-1 and IL-6] in FMS subjects (72,73). Interestingly elevated levels of IL-8 have also been reported in the peritoneal fluid of women with endometriosis (74). This finding is of some interest, as endometriosis has been linked to the development of central sensitization (75). Another study has shown elevated levels of IL-8 in the central spinal fluid of patients with cerebral lupus, another disorder commonly associated with FMS (76). Other studies have implicated IL-8 in the pathogenesis of the nerve root inflammation that occurs in response to lumbar disc herniations and also in sympathetically maintained pain (76). Interleukin 8 was originally described as a potent neutrophil chemotactic factor and is a member of C-X-C chemokine subfamily. As is the case with many of the cytokines subsequent studies have shown that it can activate a wide range of signaling molecules in a coordinate manner. Its receptor, IL-8R belongs to the family of G-protein-coupled receptors which on activation cause the release of intracellular Ca^{2+} stores with mobilization of mitogen-activated protein kinase [MAPK]. The stimulation of MAPK after G protein activation has been described as the master switch for the regulation of central sensitization (77). Members of the MAPK are a highly conserved superfamily of molecules that are a critical link in the activation of cells to different kinds of external stimuli through the modulation of gene expression. This superfamily consists of three main kinases: regulated protein kinases [ERKs], the p38 family of kinases and the c-Jun N-terminal kinases [JNKs]. Activation of p38 MAP kinase is probably of relevance to the development of central sensitization as it is activated downstream by stimulation of NMDA receptors. It is worth noting that IL-8 is synthesized by glial cells in the brain and has been shown to have a role in neuro-inflammation (78); it is released by activated glial cells with a resultant stimulation of chemokine receptors [CXCR1 and CXCR2] and cholinergic neurons activation (79). As there is increasing evidence that activation of glial cells is of relevance to pathological pain states (80,81), an increased understanding of the physiological relevance of elevated IL-8 levels will be an important area for FMS related research over the next few years.

NEUROENDOCRINE AND AUTONOMIC DYSFUNCTION

While there is now a general agreement that central sensitization is a critical component of the pain experience in FMS patients, there is still no generally accepted explanation for the symptom of fatigue. Possible reasons for fatigue in FMS include the alpha-delta sleep disturbance, cytokine induced fatigue, dysautonomia, physical deconditioning, depression, and the side effects of medications. Of course, one or several of these fatiguing factors may be present in the individual patient, but are unlikely to fully explain the total experience of fatigue. I believe an important clue to understanding fatigue in FMS patients is the strong association with stressors, both physical and mental. This suggests a central dysregulation of homeostatic mechanisms involved in the stress response. Over the past few years evidence has accumulated for dysfunction of both the neuroendocrine response to stressors and the sympatho-adrenal response to stressors. A particularly revealing study was the HPA response of FMS patients to stimulation with either low dose [1 µg] adrenocorticotrophin [ACTH] or metyrapone (82). There was a suboptimal cortisol response to ACTH in 45 percent of FMS patients and a suboptimal response of 11-deoxycortisol to metyrapone stimulation in 95 percent. A report on the basal circadian and pulsatile secretion of ACTH and cortisol in FMS patients was also consistent with a loss of HPA axis resiliency (83). Another study using a bolus injection of corticotropin releasing hormone [CRH] did not find any significant increase in either ACTH of cortisol in FMS patients compared to controls, although the plasma level of CRH following injection was significantly higher in FMS patients (23). In addition, this study found abnormalities in the hypothalamic-pituitary growth hormone axis. Basal growth hormone levels were lower in FMS patients and only increased after CRH stimulation coincidentally with a reduction of somatostatin levels. The authors concluded that these results supported the concept that hormonal dysregulation in FMS patients is primarily caused by CRH up-regulation–possibly as a response to chronic pain and stress. Another study evaluated the GH response to the stress of exhaustive exercise in FMS subjects (84). Compared to controls all FMS patients had a reduced GH response which was normalized after the subjects had been given pyridostigmine. Extensive literature indicates that a stimulation of central cholinergic tone with pyridostigmine reduces hypothalamic somatostatin tone (85-88), supporting the notion that some FMS patients have a dysregulation of the central GHRH/ somatostatin growth hormone axis. The notion that this may be due to a chronic stress response causing an up-regulation of CRH is supported by a neuroanatomical connection between CRH and somatostatin secreting neurons (89) and by animal experiments in which intra-cerebral injections of anti-somatostatin antibodies normalized a GH response that had been inhibited by a prior injection of CRH (90).

There have been several studies over the past few years that have reported a dysautonomia in FMS patients (91). The overall data suggest that many FMS patients have an increased resting sympathetic tone within an impaired acute response to stressors (92-94). Martinez-Lavin had postulated that pain in FMS is sympathetically mediated (95-98). On the other hand, heightened pain perception in FMS may be related to the inverse association between pain sensitivity and blood pressure (99-103). There are certainly important similarities between the neuroendocrine response to stress and the sympatho-adrenal response to stress in FMS patients. Exploring the interrelationships between pain and neuroendocrine/autonomic dysfunction in FMS patients should prove rewarding.

GENETIC STUDIES

There have been several studies that have reported a familial clustering of FMS patients (104-106). A recent study looking at the familial aggregation of FMS compared to rheumatoid arthritis reported that the prevalence of FMS was 6.4 percent among all relatives of probands with FMS and 18.5 percent among interviewed relatives of FMS probands. For all relatives, the estimated odds for FMS in a relative of a proband with FMS were 8.5 times the odds of FMS in a relative of a proband with rheumatoid arthritis. It was also reported that FMS strongly coaggregated with major mood disorder (107). Thus the question arises as to whether this aggregation is a result of nature or nurture. The proponents of nurture would argue that FMS is a learned pattern of maladaptive behavior and should not be considered as a distinctive disorder (108). However, there are some recent genetic linkage studies that suggest that there may be an inherited predisposition for the eventual development of FMS. Interestingly, these linkages involve monoamines such as serotonin.

Polymorphisms of the serotonin-2A receptor [HTR2A] gene have been reported to have a strong linkage to the HTR2A region in families with early age onset FMS and associated irritable bowel symptoms (abstract # 108 in Arthritis & Rheumatism Vol 48, number 9 [supplement], 2003). This gene has also been linked to attention deficit hyperactivity disorder [ADHD], seasonal affective disorder and panic disorder, but not major depression.

Serotonin transporter promoter region [5-HTTLPR] polymorphism has been considered to be a promising candidate for genetic involvement in some mood disorders owing to its role in the regulation of serotoninergic neurotransmission (109). Studies of the S/S, S/L, and L/L alleles of the 5-HTTLPR genotype in FMS have been contradictory with two showing a positive correlation with the S/S genotype (110, 111) and one negative correlation (112).

A particular variant of the HT2A receptor gene, the T102C polymorphism, has three genotypes [C/C, C/T, and T/T genotypes]. In one study of 58 FMS patients and 58 healthy controls the three genotypes were equally distributed in FMS patients compared to controls. However, There was a significant correlation between the T/T genotype and depressive symptoms and the lowest pain threshold (113). It was suggested that this polymorphism may play a role in psychiatric morbidity and FMS patients.

An intriguing study published in *Science* reported that the metabolic breakdown of monoamines by cathechol-*O*-methyltransferase [COMT] was linked to individual variability in pain sensitivity (114). There is a functional polymorphism of the COMT gene that codes the substitution of valine [*val*] by methionine [*met*] at codon 158 [*val*^{158}*met*] and results in a fourfold reduction in enzyme activity and thus influences the regulation of dopaminergic and adrenergic/noradrenergic neurotransmission. In a study of 29 healthy individuals subjected to a sustained pain stimulus [infusion of five percent hypertonic saline into the masseter muscle] it was found that subjects homozygous for the *met^158* allele of the COMT showed diminished regional μ-opioid system responses to pain compared with heterozygotes and this was paralleled by higher sensory and affective ratings of pain. Opposite effects were seen in *val^158* homozygotes. It was concluded that COMT *val^158met* polymorphism influences the individual experience of pain and may underlie variability in the physiological responses to pain and other stressors.

In a recent study of 61 FMS patients and 61 healthy subjects, three polymorphisms of the COMT gene [LL, LH, and HH] were analyzed (115). No significant differences were found between LL and LH separately, but the combination of LL and LH genotypes was more highly represented in FMS than controls. Furthermore, the HH genotype was less common in the control subjects. It was hypothesized that COMT polymorphism may underlie a genetic predisposition for the development of FMS through modulation of the adrenergic and dopaminergic systems.

MYOFASCIAL PAIN

Nearly half of the 185 myofascial pain articles cited in the NLM over the past three years were on the subject of management with botulinum toxin [BTX] injections. Overall there seems to be a general agreement that BTX injections are usually beneficial in the management of myofascial pain syndromes and migraine headaches (101,116,117). One study compared the efficacy of BTX-A with BTX-B and reported that BTX-A provided superior pain relief with a greater duration of activity (118). Furthermore, patients receiving BTX-B were more likely to have adverse events such as flu-like symptoms, injection site pain, and muscle weakness.

There is increasing interest in the mechanism of action of BTX-A, as its effect on reducing pain is seen within a few hours, whereas the reduction of muscle spasm has a latency of about one week.

This time discrepancy is difficult to reconcile with the theory that its sole mode of action is in reducing focal ischemia of muscle with the release of alogenic molecules engendered by focal sarcomere contractions (119).

Current data points to an antinociceptive effect of botulinum toxin type A that is separate from its neuromuscular activity; it seem to be related to a reduced synaptic exocytosis of other nociceptive molecules (120-122).

There does not seem to have been much progress in defining the biological basis for myofascial trigger points (123). However, there is increasing agreement that an active myofascial trigger point can be characterized by spontaneous electrical activity [SEA] that resembles endplate spike potentials (123-125). One particularly revealing study suggested that active myofascial trigger points, in comparison to latent trigger points, are characterized by a local spinal cord sensitization (126). There were several interesting studies on needle therapy for myofascial pain syndromes. One report indicated that superficial dry needling followed by active stretching was more effective than stretching alone in the inactivation of trigger points, and that stretching without prior deactivation increased trigger point sensitivity (127). There has been the clinical impression that trigger point deactivation is more effective when a local twitch response is observed; in an electrical study of myofascial trigger points in rabbits it was shown that production of a local twitch strongly correlated with an inhibition of SEA during dry needling (128).

An interesting study compared the quality of life and other measures in 33 women with FMS, 33 women with myofascial pain syndrome and 33 healthy controls (129). Overall the FMS patients had more systemic problems [fatigue, poor sleep, GI upsets, impaired vitality, numbness, and depression] than patients with uncomplicated myofascial pain syndromes. It was concluded that myofascial pain impacted mostly on physical health whereas FMS impacted on both physical and mental health.

CONCLUSIONS

From this short review of selected aspects of FMS/myofascial pain research it is evident that the past three years, since MYOPAIN '01, have witnessed several significant advances. Looking to the future I would anticipate increased research efforts on the role of peripheral pain generators, especially myofascial trigger points and cytokines, in the generation of central sensitization, with an emphasis on the role of both genetic and environmental stressors in "setting the scene" for the eventual development of fibromyalgia. A major unresolved question remains as to whether there is a central connection between heightened pain sensitivity, fatigue, and an impaired neuroendocrine/autonomic stress response. Hopefully the next three years will provide some clues to this enigma.

REFERENCES

1. Uveges JM, Parker JC, Smarr KL. Psychological symptoms in primary FMS syndrome: Relationship to pain, life stress and sleep disturbance. Arth Rheum 33: 1279-1283, 1990.

2. Boscarino JA. Diseases among men 20 years after exposure to severe stress: Implications for clinical research and medical care. Psychosom Med 59(6):605-614, 1997.

3. Amir M, Kaplan Z, Neumann L, Sharabani R, Shani N, Buskila D. Posttraumatic stress disorder, tenderness and fibromyalgia. J Psychosom Res 42(6): 607-613, 1997.

4. Cohen H, Neumann L, Haiman Y, Matar MA, Press J, Buskila D. Prevalence of post-traumatic stress disorder in FMS patients: Overlapping syndromes or post-traumatic FMS syndrome? Semin Arthritis Rheum 32(1):38-50, 2002.

5. Buskila D, Neumann L. Musculoskeletal injury as a trigger for fibromyalgia/posttraumatic fibromyalgia. Curr Rheumatol Rep 2(2):104-108, 2000.

6. Raphael KG, Natelson BH, Janal MN, Nayak S. A community-based survey of fibromyalgia-like pain complaints following the World Trade Center terrorist attacks. Pain 100(1-2):131-139, 2002.

7. Raphael KG, Janal MN, Nayak S. Comorbidity of FMS and posttraumatic stress disorder symptoms in a community sample of women. Pain Med 5(1):33-41, 2004.

8. Williams DA, Brown SC, Clauw DJ, Gendreau RM. Self-reported symptoms before and after September 11 in patients with fibromyalgia. JAMA 289(13): 1637-1638, 2003.

9. Boscarino JA, Galea S, Ahern J, Resnick H, Vlahov D. Psychiatric medication use among Manhattan residents following the World Trade Center disaster. J Trauma Stress 16(3):301-306, 2003.

10. Galea S, Resnick H, Ahern J, Gold J, Bucuvalas M, Kilpatrick D, Stuber J, Vlahov D. Posttraumatic stress disorder in Manhattan, New York City, after the September 11th terrorist attacks. J Urban Health 79(3): 340-353, 2002.

11. Galea S, Vlahov D, Resnick H, Ahern J, Susser E, Gold J, Bucuvalas M, Kilpatrick D. Trends of probable post-traumatic stress disorder in New York City after the September 11 terrorist attacks. Am J Epidemiol 158(6):514-524, 2003.

12. Pulcino T, Galea S, Ahern J, Resnick H, Foley M, Vlahov D. Posttraumatic stress in women after the September 11 terrorist attacks in New York City. J Womens Health [Larchmt] 12(8):809-820, 2003.

13. Ahern J, Galea S, Resnick H, Kilpatrick D, Bucuvalas M, Gold J, Vlahov D. Television images and psychological symptoms after the September 11 terrorist attacks. Psychiatry 65(4):289-300, 2002.

14. Volpato S, Guralnik JM, Ferrucci L, Balfour J, Chaves P, Fried LP, Guralnik JM. Cardiovascular disease, interleukin-6, and risk of mortality in older women: The women's health and aging study. Circulation Feb 20;103(7):947-953, 2001.

15. Adler GK, Kinsley BT, Hurwitz S, Mossey CJ, Goldenberg DL. Reduced hypothalamic-pituitary and sympathoadrenal responses to hypoglycemia in women with FMS syndrome. Am J Med 106(5):534-543, 1999.

16. Bremner JD, Vythilingam M, Anderson G, Vermetten E, McGlashan T, Heninger G, Rasmusson A, Southwick SM, Charney DS. Assessment of the hypothalamic-pituitary-adrenal axis over a 24-hour diurnal period and in response to neuroendocrine challenges in women with and without childhood sexual abuse and posttraumatic stress disorder. Biol Psychiatry 54(7): 710-718, 2003.

17. Kiecolt-Glaser JK, Preacher KJ, MacCallum RC, Atkinson C, Malarkey WB, Glaser R. Chronic stress and age-related increases in the pro-inflammatory cytokine IL-6. Proc Natl Acad Sci USA 100(15):9090-9095, 2003.

18. Altier N, Stewart J. The role of dopamine in the nucleus accumbens in analgesia. Life Sci 65(22): 2269-2287, 1999.

19. Altier N, Stewart J. Dopamine receptor antagonists in the nucleus accumbens attenuate analgesia induced by ventral tegmental area substance P or morphine and by nucleus accumbens amphetamine. J Pharmacol Exp Ther 285(1):208-215, 1998.

20. Wood PB. Stress and dopamine: Implications for the pathophysiology of chronic widespread pain. Med Hypotheses 62(3):420-424, 2004.

21. Senna ER, De Barros AL, Silva EO, Costa IF, Pereira LV, Ciconelli RM, Ferraz MB. Prevalence of rheumatic diseases in Brazil: A study using the COPCORD approach. J Rheumatol 31(3):594-597, 2004.

22. Carmona L, Ballina J, Gabriel R, Laffon A. The burden of musculoskeletal diseases in the general population of Spain: Results from a national survey. Ann Rheum Dis 60(11):1040-1045, 2001.

23. White KP, Nielson WR, Harth M, Ostbye T, Speechley M. Does the label "fibromyalgia" alter health status, function, and health service utilization? A prospective, within-group comparison in a community co-

hort of adults with chronic widespread pain. Arthritis Rheum 47(3):260-265, 2002.

24. White KP, Thompson J. Fibromyalgia syndrome in an Amish community: A controlled study to determine disease and symptom prevalence. J Rheumatol 30(8): 1835-1840, 2003.

25. McBeth J, Silman AJ, MacFarlane GJ. Association of widespread body pain with an increased risk of cancer and reduced cancer survival: A prospective, population-based study. Arthritis Rheum 48(6):1686-1692, 2003.

26. Vaeroy H, Helle R, Forre O, Kass E, Terenius L. Elevated CSF levels of substance P and high incidence of Raynaud phenomenon in patients with fibromyalgia: New features for diagnosis. Pain 32:21-26, 1988.

27. Russell IJ, Orr MD, Littman B, Vipraio GA, Alboukrek D, Michalek JE, Lopez Y, MacKillip F. Elevated cerebrospinal fluid levels of substance P in patients with the FMS syndrome. Arthritis Rheum 37(11): 1593-1601, 1994.

28. Liu Z, Welin M, Bragee B, Nyberg F. A high-recovery extraction procedure for quantitative analysis of substance P and opioid peptides in human cerebrospinal fluid. Peptides 21(6):853-860, 2000.

29. Vaeroy H, Nyberg F, Terenius L. No evidence for endorphin deficiency in FMS following investigation of cerebrospinal fluid [CSF] dynorphin A and Met-enkephalin-Arg6-Phe7. Pain 46(2):139-143, 1991.

30. Giovengo SL, Russell IJ, Larson AA. Increased concentrations of nerve growth factor in cerebrospinal fluid of patients with fibromyalgia. J Rheumatol 26(7): 1564-1569, 1999.

31. Staud R, Vierck CJ, Cannon RL, Mauderli AP, Price DD. Abnormal sensitization and temporal summation of second pain [wind-up] in patients with FMS syndrome. Pain 91(1-2):165-175, 2001.

32. Staud R, Cannon RC, Mauderli AP, Robinson ME, Price DD, Vierck CJ. Temporal summation of pain from mechanical stimulation of muscle tissue in normal controls and subjects with FMS syndrome. Pain 102(1-2): 87-95, 2003.

33. Lorenz J, Grasedyck K, Bromm B. Middle and long latency somatosensory evoked potentials after painful laser stimulation in patients with FMS syndrome. Electroencephalogr Clin Neurophysiol 100:165-168, 1996.

34. Granot M, Buskila D, Granovsky Y, Sprecher E, Neumann L, Yarnitsky D. Simultaneous recording of late and ultra-late pain evoked potentials in fibromyalgia. Clin Neurophysiol 112(10):1881-1887, 2001.

35. Arendt-Nielsen L, Graven-Nielsen T, Svensson P, Jensen TS. Temporal summation in muscles and referred pain areas: An experimental human study. Muscle Nerve 20(10):1311-1313, 1997.

36. Desmeules JA, Cedraschi C, Rapiti E, Baumgartner E, Finckh A, Cohen P, Dayer P, Vischer TL. Neurophysiologic evidence for a central sensitization in patients with fibromyalgia. Arthritis Rheum 48(5): 1420-1429, 2003.

37. Banica B, Petersen-Felix S, Andersen OK, Radanov BP, Villiger PM, Arendt-Nielsen L, Curatolo M. Evidence for spinal cord hypersensitivity in chronic pain after whiplash injury and in fibromyalgia. Pain 107(1-2):7-15, 2004.

38. Graven-Nielsen T, Kendall SA, Henriksson KG, Bengtsson M, Sorensen J, Johnson A, Gerdle B, Arendt-Nielsen L. Ketamine reduces muscle pain, temporal summation, and referred pain in FMS patients. Pain 85(3):483-491, 2000.

39. Sorensen J, Bengtsson A, Backman E, Henriksson KG, Bengtsson M. Pain analysis in patients with fibromyalgia: Effects of intravenous morphine, lidocaine and ketamine. Scand J Rheumatol 24:360-365, 1995.

40. Anderberg UM, Liu Z, Berglund L, Nyberg F. Elevated plasma levels of neuropeptide Y in female FMS patients. Eur J Pain 3(1):19-30, 1999.

41. Staud R, Robinson ME, Vierck CJ, Price DD. Diffuse noxious inhibitory controls [DNIC] attenuate temporal summation of second pain in normal males but not in normal females or FMS patients. Pain 101(1-2): 167-174, 2003.

42. Kosek E, Hansson P. Modulatory influence on somatosensory perception from vibration and heterotopic noxious conditioning stimulation [HNCS] in FMS patients and healthy subjects. Pain 70:41-51, 1997.

43. Gracely RH, Petzke F, Wolf JM, Clauw DJ. Functional magnetic resonance imaging evidence of augmented pain processing in fibromyalgia. Arthritis Rheum 46(5):1333-1343, 2002.

44. Cook DB, Lange G, Ciccone DS, Liu WC, Steffener J, Natelson BH. Functional imaging of pain in patients with primary fibromyalgia. J Rheumatol 31(2): 364-378, 2004.

45. Mountz JM, Bradley LA, Modell JG, Alexander RW, Triana-Alexander M, Aaron LA, Stewart KE, Alarcón GS, Mountz JD. Fibromyalgia in women. Abnormalities of regional cerebral blood flow in the thalamus and the caudate nucleus are associated with low pain threshold levels. Arthritis Rheum 38:926-938, 1995.

46. Kwiatek R, Barnden L, Tedman R, Jarrett R, Chew J, Rowe C, Pile K. Regional cerebral blood flow in fibromyalgia: Single-photon-emission computed tomography evidence of reduction in the pontine tegmentum and thalami. Arthritis Rheum 43(12):2823-2833, 2000.

47. Staud R. Fibromyalgia pain: Do we know the source? Curr Opin Rheumatol 16(2):157-163, 2004.

48. Wall PD, Woolf CJ. Muscle but not cutaneous C-afferent input produces prolonged increases in the excitability of the flexion reflex in the rat. J Physiol 356: 443-458, 1984.

49. Gowers WR. Lumbago: Its lessons and analogues. BMJ 1:117-121, 1904.

50. Bengtsson A. The muscle in fibromyalgia. Rheumatology [Oxford] 41(7):721-724, 2002.

51. Jubrias SA, Bennett RM, Klug GA. Increased incidence of a resonance in the phosphodiester region of 31P nuclear magnetic resonance spectra in the skeletal

muscle of FMS patients. Arthritis Rheum 37:801-807, 1994.

52. Arendt-Nielsen L, Graven-Nielsen T. Central sensitization in FMS and other musculoskeletal disorders. Curr Pain Headache Rep 7(5):355-361, 2003.

53. Lund E, Kendall SA, Janerot-Sjoberg B, Bengtsson A. Muscle metabolism in FMS studied by P-31 magnetic resonance spectroscopy during aerobic and anaerobic exercise. Scand J Rheumatol 32(3):138-145, 2003.

54. Sprott H, Rzanny R, Reichenbach JR, Kaiser WA, Hein G, Stein G. 31P magnetic resonance spectroscopy in fibromyalgic muscle. Rheumatology [Oxford] 39(10):1121-1125, 2000.

55. Park JH, Niermann KJ, Olsen N. Evidence for metabolic abnormalities in the muscles of patients with Fibromyalgia. Curr Rheumatol Rep 2(2):131-140, 2000.

56. Park JH, Phothimat P, Oates CT, Hernanz-Schulman M, Olsen NJ. Use of P-31 magnetic resonance spectroscopy to detect metabolic abnormalities in muscles of patients with fibromyalgia. Arthritis Rheum 41(3):406-413, 1998.

57. Vogl TJ, Sollner O, Dadashi AR, Reimers CD, Banzer D, Felix R. The value of in-vivo 31-phosphorus spectroscopy in the diagnosis of generalized muscular diseases. The clinical results and the differential diagnostic aspects. Rofo Fortschr Geb Rontgenstr Neuen Bildgeb Verfahr 162(6):455-463, 1995.

58. Waters DL, Brooks WM, Qualls CR, Baumgartner RN. Skeletal muscle mitochondrial function and lean body mass in healthy exercising elderly. Mech Ageing Dev 124(3):301-309, 2003.

59. Younkin DP, Berman P, Sladky J, Chee C, Bank W, Chance B. 31P NMR studies in Duchenne muscular dystrophy: Age-related metabolic changes. Neurology 37:165-169, 1987.

60. Graven-Nielsen T, Mense S. The peripheral apparatus of muscle pain: Evidence from animal and human studies. Clin J Pain 17(1):2-10, 2001.

61. Bennett RM, Jacobsen S. Muscle function and origin of pain in fibromyalgia. Bailliere's Clinical Rheumatology 8(4):721-746, 1994.

62. Aiken J, Bua E, Cao Z, Lopez M, Wanagat J, McKenzie D, McKiernan S. Mitochondrial DNA deletion mutations and sarcopenia. Ann N Y Acad Sci 959: 412-423, 2002.

63. Vives-Bauza C, Gamez J, Roig M, Briones P, Cervera C, Solano A, Montoya J, Andreu AL. Exercise intolerance resulting from a muscle-restricted mutation in the mitochondrial tRNA(Leu (CUN)) gene. Ann Med 33(7):493-496, 2001.

64. Kovalenko SA, Kopsidas G, Kelso JM, Linnane AW. Deltoid human muscle mtDNA is extensively rearranged in old age subjects. Biochem Biophys Res Commun 232(1):147-152, 1997.

65. Fayet G, Jansson M, Sternberg D, Moslemi AR, Blondy P, Lombes A, Fardeau M, Oldfors A. Ageing muscle: Clonal expansions of mitochondrial DNA point mutations and deletions cause focal impairment of mito-

chondrial function. Neuromuscul Disord 12(5):484-493, 2002.

66. Sprott H, Salemi S, Gay RE, Bradley LA, Alarcon GS, Oh SJ, Michel BA, Gay S. Increased DNA fragmentation and ultrastructural changes in fibromyalgic muscle fibres. Ann Rheum Dis 63(3):245-251, 2004.

67. Watkins LR, Wiertelak EP, Goehler LE, Smith KP, Martin D, Maier SF. Characterization of cytokine-induced hyperalgesia. Brain Res 654(1):15-26, 1994.

68. Vassilopoulos D, Calabrese LH. Rheumatic manifestations of hepatitis C infection. Curr Rheumatol Rep 5(3):200-204, 2003.

69. Capuron L, Hauser P, Hinze-Selch D, Miller AH, Neveu PJ. Treatment of cytokine-induced depression. Brain Behav Immun 16(5):575-580, 2002.

70. Watkins LR, Maier SF. Implications of immune-to-brain communication for sickness and pain. Proc Natl Acad Sci U S A 96(14):7710-7713, 1999.

71. Watkins LR, Milligan ED, Maier SF. Glial activation: A driving force for pathological pain. Trends Neurosci 24(8):450-455, 2001.

72. Wallace DJ, Linker-Israeli M, Hallegua D, Silverman S, Silver D, Weisman MH. Cytokines play an aetiopathogenetic role in fibromyalgia: A hypothesis and pilot study. Rheumatology [Oxford] 40(7):743-749, 2001.

73. Gur A, Karakoc M, Nas K, Remzi, Cevik, Denli A, Sarac J. Cytokines and depression in cases with fibromyalgia. J Rheumatol 292):358-361, 2002.

74. Arici A. Local cytokines in endometrial tissue: The role of interleukin-8 in the pathogenesis of endometriosis. Ann N Y Acad Sci 955:101-9 [discussion 118, 396-406], 2002.

75. Bajaj P, Bajaj P, Madsen H, Arendt-Nielsen L. Endometriosis is associated with central sensitization: A psychophysical controlled study. J Pain 4(7):372-380, 2003.

76. Trysberg E, Carlsten H, Tarkowski A. Intrathecal cytokines in systemic lupus erythematosus with central nervous system involvement. Lupus 9(7):498-503, 2000.

77. Obata K, Noguchi K. MAPK activation in nociceptive neurons and pain hypersensitivity. Life Sci 742(1):2643-2653, 2004.

78. Kwon D, Fuller AC, Palma JP, Choi IH, Kim BS. Induction of chemokines in human astrocytes by picornavirus infection requires activation of both AP-1 and NF-kappa B. Glia 45(3):287-296, 2004.

79. Puma C, Danik M, Quirion R, Ramon F, Williams S. The chemokine interleukin-8 acutely reduces Ca2+] currents in identified cholinergic septal neurons expressing CXCR1 and CXCR2 receptor mRNAs. J Neurochem 78(5):960-971, 2001.

80. Wieseler-Frank J, Maier SF, Watkins LR. Glial activation and pathological pain. Neurochem Int 45(2-3): 389-395, 2004.

81. Watkins LR, Milligan ED, Maier SF. Glial proinflammatory cytokines mediate exaggerated pain

states: implications for clinical pain. Adv Exp Med Biol 521:1-21, 2003.

82. Calis M, Gokce C, Ates F, Ulker S, Izgi HB, Demir H, Kirnap M, Sofuoglu S, Durak AC, Tutus A, Kelestimur F. Investigation of the hypothalamo-pituitary-adrenal axis [HPA] by 1 microg ACTH test and metyrapone test in patients with primary FMS syndrome. J Endocrinol Invest 27(1):42-46, 2004.

83. Crofford LJ, Young EA, Engleberg NC, Korszun A, Brucksch CB, McClure LA, Brown MB, Demitrack MA. Basal circadian and pulsatile ACTH and cortisol secretion in patients with FMS and/or chronic fatigue syndrome. Brain Behav Immun 18(4):314-325, 2004.

84. Paiva ES, Deodhar A, Jones KD, Bennett R. Impaired growth hormone secretion in FMS patients: Evidence for augmented hypothalamic somatostatin tone. Arthritis Rheum 46(5):1344-1350, 2002.

85. Corsello SM, Tofani A, Della Casa S, Sciuto R, Rota CA, Colasanti S, Bini A, Barini A, Barbarino A. Activation of cholinergic tone by pyridostigmine reverses the inhibitory effect of CRH on GHRH induced growth hormone secretion. Acta Endo (126):113-116, 1992.

86. Dinan TG, O'Keane V, Thakore J. Pyridostigmine induced growth hormone release in mania: Focus on the cholinergic/somatostatin system. Clin Endocrinol [Oxf] 40(1):93-96, 1994.

87. Giusti M, Marini G, Sessarego P, Peluffo F, Valenti S, Caratti C, Giordano G. Effect of cholinergic tone on growth hormone-releasing hormone-induced secretion of growth hormone in normal aging. Aging [Milano] 4(3):231-237, 1992.

88. Hanew K, Utsumi A, Sugawara A, Shimizu Y, Ikeda H, Abe K. The evaluation of hypothalamic somatostatin tone using pyridostigmine and thyrotropin releasing hormone in patients with acromegaly. J Endocrinol Invest 17(5):313-321, 1994.

89. Liao N, Vaudry H, Pelletier G. Neuroanatomical connections between corticotropin-releasing factor [CRF] and somatostatin [SRIF] nerve endings and thyrotropin-releasing hormone [TRH] neurons in the paraventricular nucleus of rat hypothalamus. Peptides 13(4):677-680, 1992.

90. Rivier C, Vale W. Involvement of corticotropin-releasing factor and somatostatin in stress-induced inhibition of growth hormone secretion in the rat. Endocrinology 117(6):2478-2482, 1985.

91. Raj SR, Brouillard D, Simpson CS, Hopman WM, Abdollah H. Dysautonomia among patients with fibromyalgia: A noninvasive assessment. J Rheumatol 27(11):2660-2665, 2000.

92. Martinez-Lavin M, Hermosillo AG, Mendoza C, Ortiz R, Cajigas JC, Pineda C, Nava A, Vallejo M. Orthostatic sympathetic derangement in subjects with fibromyalgia. J Rheumatol 24(4):714-718, 1997.

93. Cohen H, Neumann L, Shore M, Amir M, Cassuto Y, Buskila D. Autonomic dysfunction in patients with fibromyalgia: Application of power spectral analysis of heart rate variability [see comments]. Semin Arthritis Rheum 29(4):217-227, 2000.

94. Friederich HC, Schellberg D, Mueller K, Bieber C, Zipfel S, Eich W. Stress and autonomic dysregulation in patients with FMS syndrome. Schmerz 2004.

95. Martinez-Lavin M, Hermosillo AG. Autonomic nervous system dysfunction may explain the multisystem features of FMS [editorial. comment]. Semin Arthritis Rheum 29(4):197-199, 2000.

96. Martinez-Lavin M. Is FMS a generalized reflex sympathetic dystrophy? Clin Exp Rheumatol 19(1):1-3, 2001.

97. Martinez-Lavin M, Lopez S, Medina M, Nava A. Use of the Leeds assessment of neuropathic symptoms and signs questionnaire in patients with fibromyalgia. Semin Arthritis Rheum 32(6):407-411, 2003.

98. Martinez-Lavin M, Vidal M, Barbosa RE, Pineda C, Casanova JM, Nava A. Norepinephrine-evoked pain in fibromyalgia. A randomized pilot study [ISRCTN70707830]. BMC Musculoskelet Disord 3(1):2, 2002.

99. Absi M, Petersen KL. Blood pressure but not cortisol mediates stress effects on subsequent pain perception in healthy men and women. Pain 106(3): 285-295, 2003.

100. Campbell TS, Ditto B, Seguin JR, Sinray S, Tremblay RE. Adolescent pain sensitivity is associated with cardiac autonomic function and blood pressure over 8 years. Hypertension 41(6):1228-1233, 2003.

101. Absi M, Petersen KL, Wittmers LE. Blood pressure but not parental history for hypertension predicts pain perception in women. Pain 88(1):61-68, 2000.

102. Guasti L, Gaudio G, Zanotta D, Grimoldi P, Petrozzino MR, Tanzi F, Bertolini A, Grandi AM, Venco A. Relationship between a genetic predisposition to hypertension, blood pressure levels and pain sensitivity. Pain 82(3):311-317, 1999.

103. Okifuji A, Turk DC. Stress and psychophysiological dysregulation in patients with FMS syndrome. Appl Psychophysiol Biofeedback 27(2):129-141, 2002.

104. Pellegrino MJ, Waylonis GW, Sommer A. Familial occurrence of primary fibromyalgia. Arch Phys Med Rehabil 70:61-63, 1989.

105. Buskila D, Neumann L, Hazanov I, Carmi R. Familial aggregation in the FMS syndrome. Semin Arthritis Rheum 26:605-611, 1996.

106. Offenbaecher M, Glatzeder K, Ackenheil M. Self-reported depression, familial history of depression and FMS [FM], and psychological distress in patients with FM. Z Rheumatol 57 (Suppl 2):94-96, 1998.

107. Arnold LM, Hudson JI, Hess EV, Ware AE, Fritz DA, Auchenbach MB, Starck LO, Keck PE Jr. Family study of fibromyalgia. Arthritis Rheum 50(3):944-952, 2004.

108. Ehrlich GE. Pain is real. FMS isn't. J Rheumatol 30(8):1666-1667, 2003.

109. Owens MJ, Nemeroff CB. Role of serotonin in the pathophysiology of depression: Focus on the serotonin transporter. Clin Chem 40:288-295, 1994.

110. Cohen H, Buskila D, Neumann L, Ebstein RP. Confirmation of an association between FMS and serotonin transporter promoter region [5-HTTLPR] polymorphism, and relationship to anxiety-related personality traits. Arthritis Rheum 46(3):845-847, 2002.

111. Offenbaecher M, Bondy B, de Jonge S, Glatzeder K, Kruger M, Schoeps P, Ackenheil M. Possible association of FMS with a polymorphism in the serotonin transporter gene regulatory region. Arthritis Rheum 42(11):2482-2488, 1999.

112. Gursoy S. Absence of association of the serotonin transporter gene polymorphism with the mentally healthy subset of FMS patients. Clin Rheumatol 21(3): 194-197, 2002.

113. Gursoy S, Erdal E, Herken H, Madenci E, Alasehirli B. Association of T102C polymorphism of the 5-HT2A receptor gene with psychiatric status in FMS syndrome. Rheumatol Int 21(2):58-61, 2001.

114. Zubieta JK, Heitzeg MM, Smith YR, Bueller JA, Xu K, Xu Y, Koeppe RA, Stohler CS, Goldman D. COMT val158met genotype affects mu-opioid neurotransmitter responses to a pain stressor. Science 299(5610):1240-1243, 2003.

115. Gursoy S, Erdal E, Herken H, Madenci E, Alasehirli B, Erdal N. Significance of catechol-O-methyltransferase gene polymorphism in FMS syndrome. Rheumatol Int 23(3):104-107, 2003.

116. De Andres J, Cerda-Olmedo G, Valia JC, Monsalve V, Lopez A, Minguez A. Use of botulinum toxin in the treatment of chronic myofascial pain. Clin J Pain 19(4):269-275, 2003.

117. Dodick D, Blumenfeld A, Silberstein SD. Botulinum neurotoxin for the treatment of migraine and other primary headache disorders. Clin Dermatol 22(1): 76-81, 2004.

118. Lang AM. A preliminary comparison of the efficacy and tolerability of botulinum toxin serotypes A and B in the treatment of myofascial pain syndrome: A retrospective, open-label chart review. Clin Ther 25(8): 2268-2278, 2003.

119. Mense S. Neurobiological basis for the use of botulinum toxin in pain therapy. J Neurol 251 (Suppl 1):7-17, 2004.

120. Aoki KR. Evidence for antinociceptive activity of botulinum toxin type A in pain management. Headache 43 (Suppl 1):S9-15, 2003.

121. Kramer HH, Angerer C, Erbguth F, Schmelz M, Birklein F. Botulinum Toxin A reduces neurogenic flare but has almost no effect on pain and hyperalgesia in human skin. J Neurol 250(2):188-193, 2003.

122. Dolly O. Synaptic transmission: Inhibition of neurotransmitter release by botulinum toxins. Headache 43 (Suppl 1):S16-24, 2003.

123. Hong CZ. New trends in myofascial pain syndrome. Zhonghua Yi Xue Za Zhi [Taipei] 65(11): 501-512, 2002.

124. Simons DG, Hong CZ, Simons LS. Endplate potentials are common to midfiber myofacial trigger points. Am J Phys Med Rehabil 81(3):212-222, 2002.

125. Rivner MH. The neurophysiology of myofascial pain syndrome. Curr Pain Headache Rep 5(5):432-440, 2001.

126. Audette JF, Wang F, Smith H. Bilateral activation of motor unit potentials with unilateral needle stimulation of active myofascial trigger points. Am J Phys Med Rehabil 83(5):368-74, quiz, 2004.

127. Edwards J, Knowles N. Superficial dry needling and active stretching in the treatment of myofascial pain–A randomised controlled trial. Acupunct Med 21(3):80-86, 2003.

128. Chen JT, Chung KC, Hou CR, Kuan TS, Chen SM, Hong CZ. Inhibitory effect of dry needling on the spontaneous electrical activity recorded from myofascial trigger spots of rabbit skeletal muscle. Am J Phys Med Rehabil 80(10):729-735, 2001.

129. Tuzun EH, Albayrak G, Eker L, Sozay S, Daskapan A. A comparison study of quality of life in women with FMS and myofascial pain syndrome. Disabil Rehabil 26(4):198-202, 2004.

Mechanisms of the Transition
from Acute to Chronic Pain

Walter Zieglgänsberger

Objectives: Chronic pain states may arise from synaptic and cellular plasticity in a variety of distinct systems. Novel compounds and new regimes for drug treatment to prevent activity-dependent long-term changes are emerging.

Methods: Novel electrophysiological, molecular, and cellular biological techniques have changed the face of pain research by detailing the multiplicity of transducing and suppressive systems which involve neuronal and hormonal systems acting in concert to help the individual to cope with pain.

Results: Synaptic excitation following nociceptor activation triggers sets of neuronal events which extend over a time frame ranging from milliseconds to hours, days, or weeks. While the earliest short-term responses are reflected in rapid changes of neuronal discharge activity, the long-term changes most commonly require alterations in gene expression. Immediate-early-genes code for transcription factors and participate as third messengers in the late phase of the stimulus transcription cascade. Similar neuroplastic changes take place in other components of the pain matrix.

Conclusions: "Memory traces" of pain are not necessarily permanent but can gradually diminish spontaneously or can be reversed by adequate therapeutic intervention. In the absence of reinforcement, the behavioral responses resulting from aversive memories will gradually diminish to be finally extinct. In a recent study we showed that in mice that were deficient in cannabinoid receptor 1 the extinction of aversive memory was impaired (Marsicano et al., Nature 418, 2002).

Walter Zieglgänsberger, Prof. Dr. med., is affiliated with the Max Planck Institute of Psychiatry, Munich, Germany.

[Haworth co-indexing entry note]: "Mechanisms of the Transition from Acute to Chronic Pain." Zieglgänsberger, Walter. Co-published simultaneously in *Journal of Musculoskeletal Pain* [The Haworth Medical Press, an imprint of The Haworth Press, Inc.] Vol. 12, No. 3/4, 2004, p. 13; and: *Soft Tissue Pain Syndromes: Clinical Diagnosis and Pathogenesis* [ed: Dieter E. Pongratz, Siegfried Mense, and Michael Spaeth] The Haworth Medical Press, an imprint of The Haworth Press, Inc., 2004, p. 13. Single or multiple copies of this article are available for a fee from The Haworth Document Delivery Service [1-800-HAWORTH, 9:00 a.m. - 5:00 p.m. [EST]. E-mail address: docdelivery@haworthpress.com].

Available online at http://www.haworthpress.com/web/JMP
doi:10.1300/J094v12n03_02

New Aspects of Myofascial Trigger Points: Etiological and Clinical

David G. Simons

SUMMARY. Objectives: To identify important new developments in our understanding of the nature and clinical characteristics of myofascial trigger points [TrPs].

Findings: Recent research studies reinforce the credibility of three key features of an integrated hypothesis that is designed to explain the pathophysiology of TrPs: increased acetylcholine effect, increased muscle-fiber tension, and local release of sensitizing substances. Electromyographic studies of TrPs support an increased acetylcholine effect that produces endplate noise. Nine histological studies of animal and human subjects identify features that indicate abnormally increased muscle-fiber tension and help to account for the taut bands observed clinically. Microdialysis studies by Jay Shah, MD and colleagues at the National Institutes of Health compared, in nine subjects, the findings in active TrPs to findings in latent TrPs and in normal muscles [nine examinations]. They found a significantly reduced pressure pain threshold and pH at the three active TrPs. In active TrPs, seven pain-related substances were significantly increased: substance P, calcitonin gene-related peptide, bradykinin, serotonin, norepinephrine, tumor necrosis factor, and interleukin-1β. Using shockwave generators, Wolfgang Bauermeister, MD located active TrPs in the gluteus medius and/or gluteus minimus muscles in all of 114 patients with sciatica. In another study, treatment of idiopathic low back pain with piezoelectric generated shockwaves resulted in 80 percent reduction of pain in 15 of 20 patients after 10 treatments. Treatment with electrohydraulic shockwaves reduced the pain 85 percent in 18 of 20 patients after six treatments.

Conclusions: The microdialysis findings in TrPs help to validate the integrated hypothesis and to explain the painfulness of TrPs. Either an electrohydraulic or piezoelectric shockwave device can be used to locate and treat TrPs. Clinically, the electrohydraulic method seems preferable. *[Article copies available for a fee from The Haworth Document Delivery Service: 1-800-HAWORTH. E-mail address: <docdelivery@haworthpress.com> Website: <http://www.HaworthPress.com> © 2004 by The Haworth Press, Inc. All rights reserved.]*

KEYWORDS. Myofascial pain, trigger points, prevalence, diagnosis, microdialysis, shockwave

INTRODUCTION

Before exploring what is new in the field of myofascial trigger points [TrPs] let us first consider where they fit into the big picture. Despite the fact that an increasing number of clinicians and scientists believe that most of the common enigmatic unexplained musculoskeletal pain comes from TrPs, mainstream medicine has yet to accept or incorporate them as an integral part

David G. Simons, MD, MS, DSc [Hon.], is Clinical Professor [Voluntary], Department of Rehabilitation Medicine, Emory University, Atlanta, GA, USA.

[Haworth co-indexing entry note]: "New Aspects of Myofascial Trigger Points: Etiological and Clinical." Simons, David G. Co-published simultaneously in *Journal of Musculoskeletal Pain* [The Haworth Medical Press, an imprint of The Haworth Press, Inc.] Vol. 12, No. 3/4, 2004, pp. 15-21; and: *Soft Tissue Pain Syndromes: Clinical Diagnosis and Pathogenesis* [ed: Dieter E. Pongratz, Siegfried Mense, and Michael Spaeth] The Haworth Medical Press, an imprint of The Haworth Press, Inc., 2004, pp. 15-21. Single or multiple copies of this article are available for a fee from The Haworth Document Delivery Service [1-800-HAWORTH, 9:00 a.m. - 5:00 p.m. [EST]. E-mail address: docdelivery@haworthpress.com].

Available online at http://www.haworthpress.com/web/JMP
doi:10.1300/J094v12n03_03

of its teaching, research, and practice. Several factors that are now starting to clear up help to account for the slow progress.

It is becoming increasingly clear that, although the core of TrPs lies in skeletal muscle, all branches of the nervous system and several endocrine systems interact with them; TrPs are very complex. Three factors appear to be critical. 1. There is no generally accepted pathophysiology to account for the symptoms of TrPs, which thwarts the establishment of authoritative diagnostic criteria, the lack of which discourages research concerning their pathophysiology. 2. At present, there is no recognized laboratory test or imaging technique to serve as a diagnostic gold standard for TrPs. The diagnosis can be made only by history and physical examination. 3. In the absence of an established gold-standard diagnostic test, appropriate specific diagnostic criteria remain controversial and unresolved. This is in part because clinicians depend heavily on the history as well as the physical examination but interrater reliability studies to date have addressed only the physical examination. These interrater reliability studies make it clear that for many clinicians it takes training and much experience to develop adequate skill for diagnostic reliability [and for therapeutic competence]. Agreement on diagnostic criteria is also confounded by the many variations in structure and accessibility of some 500 individual muscles; no one examination applies to all muscles.

ETIOLOGY

Currently, the only proposed etiology of TrPs that effectively explains their most widely recognized clinical features (1) is the integrated hypothesis (2-4). This hypothesis postulates three essential features that relate to one another in a positive feedback cycle [Figure 1] that is self-perpetuating once it is started but can be interrupted at several points in the cycle in a number of ways. There is now substantial evidence for the presence of three key pathophysiological features of TrPs, but the pathways between them are not as well established.

The three features are increased acetylcholine release at the neuromuscular junction [motor endplate], increased muscle-fiber tension of

FIGURE 1. Three essential pathophysiological features of myofascial trigger points and their relationship in a positive feedback cycle.

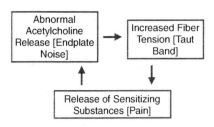

fibers passing through the TrP that produces a palpable taut band, and the presence of sensitizing substances in the muscle tissue of the TrP that can produce pain.

Acetylcholine Release

The concept that increased acetylcholine release is a characteristic feature of TrP pathophysiology is based on electrodiagnostic evidence. Reviews of basic physiology research established that the increased electrical activity at the motor endplate that is characteristic of endplate noise is associated with greatly increased release of acetylcholine transmitter (5,3). Two independent studies showed that endplate noise is significantly related to TrPs (6,7). However, increased release of acetylcholine packets is not the only way increased endplate noise could be generated. If some other mechanism such as an immune system reaction were to block the normally prompt inactivation of acetylcholine by cholinesterase within the synaptic cleft, the acetylcholine receptors in the postjunctional membrane would continue to produce excessive numbers of miniature endplate potentials [endplate noise]. The blockage of cholinesterase has been used as an experimental tool to study the effects of increased acetylcholine release.

Calcitonin gene-related peptide inhibits the expression of cholinesterase in vertebrate experiments (8). This would allow more acetylcholine to affect receptors in the postjunctional membrane producing an effect comparable to increased release of acetylcholine. The peptide also can induce expression of the acetylcholine receptor (9) that would also increase the number of miniature endplate potentials.

Increased Fiber Tension

The specific mechanisms responsible for the taut band are not yet clear. Clinically, those who successfully diagnose and treat TrPs consider the taut band an essential feature of TrPs. Seven of the eight studies that evaluated interrater reliability for identifying TrPs included identification of a taut band as one of the criteria tested. Both human and animal biopsy studies reveal several kinds of evidence of increased tension in some individual muscle fibers. See Table 1. In some cases, all one sees are torn muscle fibers and electron microscopic evidence of disrupted contractile elements. Sometimes local regions of hypercontracted fibers are observed as contraction knots or contraction discs that

TABLE 1. Summary of Biopsy Studies Relating to Myofascial Trigger Points.

Article	Subject	Situation	Microscopy
Blackman et al. 1973 (10)	mouse/rat diaphragm	decamethonium +3 other choline agonists	electron microscopic: "crimps"
Simons & Stolov 1976 (11)	dog, gracilis & sartorius muscle	natural TrPs in rather old animals	light microscopic: trichrome stain, "contraction knots"
Hudson et al. 1978 (12)	rats–extensor digitorum longus	neostigmine methyl sulfate, an anti-cholinesterase	electron microscopic: "localized subjunctional super contraction" of sarcomeres
Duxson et al. 1985 (13)	rats–biceps femoris muscle	DFP-diisopropyl-fluorophosphate–a cholinesterase inhibitor	electron microscopic: super contracture under endplate
Mense et al. 2003 (14)	rats–gastrocnemius muscle	muscle stimulation and DFP-diisopropyl fluorophosphate–a cholinesterase inhibitor	light microscopic: contraction discs, disrupted fibers
Reitinger et al. 1996 (15)	human gluteus medius and minimus	biopsies of myogelotic nodules at TrP locations in patients	light and electron microscopic: large round fibers
Windisch et al. 1999 (16)	human trapezius and gluteal muscles	post mortem biopsies of myogelotic areas [like trigger points]	light microscopic: large round fibers, local fiber degenerative changes
Pongratz et al. 2004 (17)	human	biopsies of TrPs in patients	electron microscopic: locally shortened sarcomas
Devlikamova et al. 2004 (18)	human trapezius muscle	myofascial trigger zone of patient	destruction of cytoskeletal protein, abnormal mitochondria

TrP = myofascial trigger point

would increase tension in that fiber. These local regions of severely shortened sarcomeres characteristically have adjacent regions of compensatory lengthening of the sarcomeres in that fiber, which would further increase tension in that fiber because of the elastic resistance of sarcomeres to passive stretch, especially with elongation beyond resting length. These observations help to explain the increased muscle tension in muscles that have TrPs.

Several studies of mammalian muscle in animals have demonstrated that a spindle-shaped region of hypercontracted sarcomeres in a muscle fiber under the motor endplate can develop in response to effectively increasing exposure of the postjunctional membrane to acetylcholine. Blackman (10), in 1973, produced 'crimps' by applying choline agonists. Simons and Stolov (11), in 1975, reported contraction knots in TrPs of dogs. Two other investigations (12,13) demonstrated super contracted fibers under the endplate with a cholinesterase inhibitor. Mense et al. (14) observed contraction discs with a cholinesterase inhibitor and electrical stimulation of the muscle. None of the four biopsy reports in humans (15-18) identified contraction knots, but the first two identified large round muscle fibers, as reported in the 1975 dog study. The first TrP study in humans (15) did not include longitudinal sections that are required to see contraction knots. The third (17) reported primarily electron microscopic findings. All saw evidence of increased muscle tension and tissue distress. Biopsy studies in humans that concentrate on the presence of regionally shortened sarcomeres and any other cause for abnormal tension of muscle fibers are urgently needed to clarify the source[s] of the increased tension of bundles of fibers that constitute palpable taut bands.

Sensitizing Substances

The algogenic characteristics of many substances that cause muscle pain have been described in detail in the book, *Muscle Pain* (19). A recent, objective, in-depth review of the literature on TrPs observed that to date no experiment had demonstrated sensitizing substances at TrPs that were postulated by the integrated hypothesis. That has now changed, as described below.

CLINICAL DEVELOPMENTS

Trigger-Point Tissue Milieu

Jay Shah, MD, Department of Rehabilitation Medicine, Clinical Center of the National Institutes of Health and colleagues (20) described a study of the tissue milieu in TrPs of nine subjects [three normal subjects without symptoms or evidence of TrPs, three with latent TrPs, and three with active TrPs]. They used a novel [and most remarkable] acupuncture-size microdialysis needle to sample both normal tissue and TrPs in upper trapezius muscles. The acupuncture needle contained in- and out-delivery tubes that ended at a dialyzer membrane set 0.2 mm from the open tip of the needle.

Results are summarized in Table 2. Active TrP sites had lower pain pressure thresholds than latent or normal sites [$P < 0.08$] and were also more pressure sensitive than the latent sites. The initial pH was lower at active sites than at the other two sites [$P < 0.03$]. Overall, the initial amounts for each of the other substances at active sites was greater than at the other two sites [at least $P < 0.01$]. At five minutes, peak levels of substance P and calcitonin gene-related peptide differed significantly in all three groups [active > latent > control sites, $P < 0.02$].

TABLE 2. Comparison of the Relative Amounts of Possible Algogenic Substances Sampled by Microdialysis from Three Active Myofascial Trigger Points Compared to Samples from Three Latent Trigger Points and from Three Control Sites.

Measurement	Active TrPs compared with latent TrPs and normal muscles
Pressure Pain Threshold [PPT]	↓ $P < 0.08$
pH	↓ $P < 0.03$
Substance P [SP]	↑ $P < 0.01$
Calcitonin Gene-Related Peptide [CGRP]	↑ $P < 0.01$
Bradykinin	↑ $P < 0.01$
Serotonin	↑ $P < 0.01$
Norepinephrine	↑ $P < 0.01$
Tumor Necrosis Factor [TNF-α]	↑ $P < 0.001$
Interleukin [IL-1β]	↑ $P < 0.001$

TrPs = trigger points
PPT = pressure pain threshold
CGRP = calcitonin gene-related peptide
TNF-α = tumor necrosis factor-alpha
IL-1β = interleukin-beta

In conclusion, the significant differences in all of these substances between normal muscle tissue and trigger point sites demonstrate for the first time that TrPs have a demonstrable and remarkably complex histopathology. This histopathology verifies the existence of TrPs as a significant clinical entity and also confirms a major step of the integrated hypothesis related to TrPs. There is now a solid experimental basis for the pain that is characteristic of TrPs. The significant histochemical difference in the findings at latent and active TrPs provides a measurable substantiation of the important clinical distinction between the two.

Shockwave Device

Although shockwave therapy for lithotripsy of renal calculi is well known, its application to TrPs is a recent and promising development. The usefulness of shockwave devices for identifying TrPs depends on the kind of device used (21). Devices using radial pressure waves that lack focus are seriously limited because of rapid decay of the pressure wave with distance from the applicator.

The waves generated by the piezoelectric device are more sharply focused than the waves generated by the electrohydraulic system. The depth of the focal point in the tissue is also adjustable, making piezoelectric devices more accurate for locating TrPs, especially in deeply placed muscles.

On the other hand, hydroelectric devices generate shockwaves with lower peak maximum pressure and a larger area of coverage. This permits more rapid screening of muscle for TrPs, but with less precise localization (21).

Bauermeister (22) compared the effectiveness of piezoelectric and electro-hydraulic types of shockwave emitters for identifying active TrPs in the gluteus medius and gluteus minimus muscles of 114 subjects with chronic sciatica-type pain that had been unresponsive to conventional treatments. Fifty-seven subjects were examined with each type of emitter. The total energy of emission during each test shock was adjusted to produce a pain level of 60 on a visual analog scale of 100. The average energy required from the piezoelectric emitter was 0.82 mJ/mm^2, and from the electro-hydraulic emitter was 0.266 mJ/mm^2 [only 1/3 as much].

In every case, an active TrP was located by eliciting a pain familiar to the subject. Although this degree of stimulation would likely cause referred pain from latent TrPs, that pain should not be familiar to the subject.

In another study (23), Bauermeister compared diagnostic and treatment experience with two kinds of shockwaves. Each type was applied to half of 40 subjects with chronic idiopathic low back pain unresponsive to conventional treatment. The results are presented in Table 3. For diagnosis and treatment of TrPs, the electro-hydraulic device was preferable in every way. It caused the subject less pain during testing, made it easier to locate active TrPs, elicited local twitch responses, and also provided more relief from low back pain with fewer treatments. Both devices were remarkably more effective therapeutically than previous conventional treatments on those patients and are compared in Table 3. The piezoelectric shock is concentrated in a much smaller region that makes it more useful for precise localization of a TrP, especially for research purposes.

Diagnosis

Six of eight studies to test interrater reliability of examiners for the identification of TrPs by physical examination criteria alone concluded that the results were unsatisfactory for clinical purposes. Comparison of these six

TABLE 3. Clinical Characteristics of Two Kinds of Shockwave Generators, Piezoelectric and Electrohydraulic, that Were Compared in Two Similar Groups of 20 Patients with Idiopathic Low Back Pain Unresponsive to Conventional Therapy. For Therapeutic Purposes, the Electrohydraulic Type Was More Satisfactory.

Diagnostic and treatment experience	Piezoelectric N = 20	Electrohydraulic N = 20
Pain at TrP during testing	greater	less
Locating an active TrP	more difficult	easier
Eliciting a local twitch response	not responsive	responsive
80 percent reduction in pain [VAS]	15 of 20 patients [75 percent] after 10 treatments	
85 percent reduction in pain [VAS]		18 of 20 patients [90 percent] after 6 treatments

N = number
TrP = myofascial trigger point
VAS = visual analog scale

studies (24-29) with the two studies reporting good results (24,30) indicates that the poor results may be due to a number of commonly overlooked realities: 1. for many clinicians, the necessary skill and specificity of examination technique requires adequate training and extensive clinical experience; 2. some muscles are considerably more difficult to examine reliably than others and some require modifications of the examination technique; 3. the patient history is an important part of the diagnostic process that is bypassed with this physical examination-only approach.

A considerable variety of diagnostic examinations were tested as indicative of TrPs. Repeatedly, recognized elicited pain [indicative of an active TrP] was one of the most reliable examinations. The local twitch response was the least reliable, especially in deeper muscles, but is a highly specific indicator of a TrP. Since a local twitch response is probably not an essential part of the pathophysiology of TrPs, it may be considered a valuable diagnostic finding, but not essential. On the other hand, although the presence of a palpable taut band was usually reported to be the next least reliable examination, it does appear to be an essential component of TrP pathology and is considered by skilled clinicians to be one of the most important diagnostic findings. Seven of the eight interrater reliability studies included the taut band as a diagnostic examination. It now appears that the minimum essential diagnostic criteria for a latent TrP is a tender spot in a taut band (31) from which referred pain can be elicited. It also appears that an active TrP is a TrP that meets latent criteria and is one from which pain can be elicited that is familiar [recognized as one the subject has experienced lately].

Interactions of Myofascial Trigger Points

Although the core of TrPs appears to be a neuromuscular dysfunction of skeletal muscle, TrPs are incredibly complex and interact with all major components of the central nervous system, with the endocrine systems, and with the immune system. For this reason, it can be a serious mistake to consider the TrP in isolation. Trigger Points often occur in clusters involving regional function. Dr. Karel Lewit has recognized the tendency of TrPs to appear in chains of functionally related muscles with emphasis on the deep stabilizers of the lower torso, especially in the diaphragm and pelvic floor muscles (32). The importance of the core stabilizer muscles is now becoming recognized, but the diaphragm is often overlooked (33). The surprising observation that TrPs in these core muscles are so commonly an important part of headache warns us to be concerned with the big picture as well as with the TrPs of individual muscles. Chronicity of TrPs often results from failure to identify and correct important perpetuating factors. We apparently have yet to realize the full depth and extent of the complexity of TrPs.

CONCLUSIONS

Several major roadblocks to the acceptance and recognition of TrPs as a neuromuscular disease by mainstream medicine appear to be starting to crumble. The critical issue of what constitutes the essential features of TrPs and what is required to identify them with adequate reliability is being approached from several directions. The basis for a more objective diagnostic tool, shockwave technology, may be in sight. The controversial issue of the pathophysiology of TrPs is accumulating an increasingly solid experimental base on several fronts. Shockwave technology offers a promising new way of treating TrPs. Several lines of evidence emphasize the remarkable and daunting complexity of TrPs. There will always remain the very important challenge of identifying and correcting the structural and medical perpetuating factors that cause and sustain chronicity.

REFERENCES

1. Simons DG: Understanding effective treatments of myofascial trigger points. J of Bodywork and Movement Therapies 6(2):81-88, 2002.

2. Simons DG, Travell JG, Simons LS: Travell and Simons' Myofascial Pain and Dysfunction: The Trigger Point Manual. Vol 1, Second Edition. Lippincott Williams & Wilkins. Baltimore, 1999, pp. 57-78.

3. Simons DG: Review of enigmatic TrPs as a common cause of enigmatic musculoskeletal pain and dysfunction. J Electromyog Kinesiol 14(1):95-107, 2004.

4. Simons DG, Mense S: Diagnose und Therapie myofaszialer Triggerpunkte [Diagnosis and Therapy of Myofascial Trigger Points] Der Schmerz 17(6):419-424, 2003.

5. Simons DG: Do endplate noise and spikes arise from normal motor endplates? Am J Phys Med Rehabil 80(2):134-140, 2001.

6. Couppé C, Midttun A, Hilden J, Jørgensen U, Oxholm P, Fuglsang-Frederiksen A: Spontaneous needle electromyographic activity in myofascial trigger points in the infraspinatus muscle: A blinded assessment. J Musculoske Pain 9(3):7-16, 2001.

7. Simons DG, Hong C-Z, Simons LS: Endplate potentials are common to midfiber myofascial trigger points. Am J Phys Med Rehabil 81(3):212-222, March 2002.

8. Rossi SG, Dickerson IM. Rotundo RI: Localization of the calcitonin gene-related peptide receptor complex at the vertebrate neuromuscular junction and its role in regulating acetylcholinesterase expression. J Biol Chem 278(27)Jul 4:24994-5000, 2003.

9. New H, Mudge A: Calcitonin gene-related peptide regulates muscle acetylcholine receptor synthesis. Nature 323:809-811, 1986.

10. Blackman JG, Hopkins WG, Milne RJ, Peterson DW: Supercontracture at endplates of mammalian muscle fibers caused by decamethonium and related agonists. Proceedings of the University of Otago Medical School 56(3):71-72, 1973.

11. Simons DG, Stolov WC: Microscopic features and transient contraction of palpable bands in canine muscle. Am J Phys Med 55:65-88, 1976.

12. Hudson CS, Rash JE, Tiedt TN, Albuquerque EX: Neostigmine-induced alterations at the mammalian neuromuscular junction. II. Ultrastructure. J Pharmacol Exp Therapeutics 205(2):340-356, 1978.

13. Duxson MJ, Vrbova G: Inhibition of acetylcholinesterase accelerates axon terminal withdrawal at the developing rat neuromuscular junction. J Neurophysiol 14:337-363, 1985.

14. Mense S, Simons DG, Hoheisel U, Quenzer B: Lesions of rat skeletal muscle following local block of acetylcholinesterase and neuromuscular stimulation. J Appl Physiol 94:2494-2501, 2003 (on-line version available PubMed ID #12576409 dated 7 Feb 2003).

15. Reitinger A, Radner H, Tilscher H, Hanna M, Windisch A, Feigl W: Morphologische Untersuchung an Triggerpunkten [Morphologic study of trigger points]. Manuelle Medizin 34:256-262, 1996.

16. Windisch A, Reitinger A, Traxler H, Radner H, Neumayer C, Feigl W, Firbas W: Morphology and histochemistry of myogelosis. Clinical Anatomy 12:266-271, 1999.

17. Pongratz D, Vorgerd M, Schoser BGH: Scientific aspects and clinical signs of muscle pain. J Musculoske Pain 12(Supplement 9):9, 2004.

18. Devlikamova FL, Polygalova OO, Rogozhin AA: Ultrastructure changes in trapezius muscle in myofascial pain syndrome. J Musculoske Pain 12(Supplement 9):16, 2004 (Abstract).

19. Mense S, Simons DG, Russell IJ: Muscle Pain: Its Nature, Diagnosis, and Treatment. Lippincott, Williams & Wilkins, Philadelphia, 2001.

20. Shah JP, Phillips T, Danoff J, Gerber L: Novel microanalytical technique distinguishes three clinically distinct groups: (1) subjects without pain and without a myofascial trigger point; (2) subjects without pain with a myofascial trigger point; (3) subjects with pain and a myofascial trigger point. Am J Phys Med Rehabil 83 (3):231, 2004 (Abstract).

21. Schultheiss R, Bauermeister W: Shockwave parameters and their potential influence of the diagnosis of myofascial pain. J Musculoske Pain 12(Supplement 9): 36, 2004 (Abstract).

22. Bauermeister W: The diagnosis and treatment of myofascial trigger points using shockwaves. J Musculoske Pain 12(Supplement 9):13, 2004 (Abstract).

23. Bauermeister W: The diagnosis and treatment of myofascial trigger points using shockwaves in patients with "idiopathic" low back pain. J Musculoske Pain 12(Supplement 9):13, 2004 (Abstract).

24. Gerwin RD, Shannon S, Hong C-Z, et al.: Inter-rater reliability in myofascial trigger point examination. Pain 69:65-73, 1997.

25. Hsieh C-Y, Hong C-Z, Adams AH, et al. Inter-examiner reliability of the palpation of trigger points in the trunk and lower limb muscles. Arch Phys Med Rehabil. 81:258-264, 2000.

26. Lew PC, Lewis, J, Story I. Inter-therapist reliability in locating latent myofascial trigger points using palpation. Manual Therapy 2(2):87-90, 1997.

27. Nice DA, Riddle DL, Lamb RL, et al.: Intertester reliability of judgments of the presence of trigger points in patients. Arch Phys Med Rehabil 73:893-898, 1992.

28. Njoo KH, Van der Does E. The occurrence and inter-rater reliability of myofascial trigger points in the quadratus lumborum and gluteus medius: A prospective study in non-specific low back pain patients and controls in general practice. Pain 58:317-323, 1994.

29. Wolfe F, Simons D, Fricton J, et al.: The fibromyalgia and myofascial pain syndromes: A preliminary study of tender points and trigger points in persons with fibromyalgia, myofascial pain syndrome, and no disease. The Journal of Rheumatology 19:944-951, 1992

30. Sciotti VM, Mittak VL, DiMarco L, et al.: Clinical precision of myofascial trigger point location in the trapezius muscle. Pain 93:259-266, 2001.

31. Gerwin RD, Dommerholt J: Trigger point inactivation and the criteria for trigger point identification. J Musculoske Pain 12(Supplement 9):47, 2004 (Abstract).

32. Lewit K: Incidence and possible role of myofascial trigger points in migraine. J Musculoske Pain 12(Supplement 9):31, 2004 (Abstract).

33. Akuthota V, Nadler SF: Core strengthening. Arch Phys Med Rehabil 85 (S1):S86-S92, 2004.

Differential Diagnosis of Trigger Points

Robert Gerwin

SUMMARY. Objective: A number of medical and structural conditions produce muscular pain associated with myofascial trigger points [TrPs]. These conditions should be considered when evaluating a patient with muscle pain.

Thesis: Myofascial pain syndrome is characterized by regional or widespread myalgia with muscle TrPs. Trigger points are also common in fibromyalgia. The TrP is a physical sign that occurs in a variety of myalgic conditions. Acute or chronic muscle stress creates an "energy crisis" that can result in a TrP. A muscle-related nociceptive stimulation of the peripheral and central nervous system results in hypersensitivity. Both mechanical and systemic medical disorders stress muscle. Mechanical problems can be structural or postural. Static [postural] or acute [trauma] muscle overload occurs in mechanical disorders which results in physical and biochemical changes including hypoxia and ischemia, and neuromuscular junction dysfunction. Delayed onset muscle pain is seen in unaccustomed eccentric exercise. Post-laminectomy and failed spinal fusions are causes of myofascial pain syndrome. Systemic medical disorders can result in diffuse TrP-related myalgia, though the mechanism may be unclear. Systemic medical disorders that cause TrP-related pain include connective tissue disorders [hypermobility syndrome and polymyalgia rheumatica], hypothyroidism, vitamin B_{12} insufficiency, and infectious diseases [Lyme disease and parasitic infection]. Drug induced myalgia ['statin' drugs, propoxyphene, and penicillamine] and myalgic encephalomyelitis/chronic fatigue syndrome, neurogenic myalgia in radiculopathy or nerve entrapment, and viscerosomatic pain syndromes are all important causes.

Conclusion: Trigger points pain can have many different causes that must be identified and treated specifically. *[Article copies available for a fee from The Haworth Document Delivery Service: 1-800-HAWORTH. E-mail address: <docdelivery@haworthpress.com> Website: <http://www.HaworthPress. com> © 2004 by The Haworth Press, Inc. All rights reserved.]*

KEYWORDS. Myalgia, myofascial pain syndrome, trigger points

MYALGIA

The term myalgia refers to painful or tender muscle, without distinction as to whether the pain or tenderness is from fibromyalgia [FMS] or myofascial pain syndrome [MPS]. Inflammatory myalgias like polymyositis and dermatomyositis present problems quite different from those of MPS and FMS, and will not be discussed here. The focus of this discussion will be on those conditions that must be considered when encountering patients with non-inflammatory muscle tenderness and pain. These conditions can be conveniently divided into mechanical causes of muscle pain, and non-mechanical or medical causes of muscle pain.

Mechanical causes of myalgia can be subdivided into ergonomic, structural, and postural

Robert Gerwin, MD, is affiliated with the Johns Hopkins University, Baltimore, MD, USA.

[Haworth co-indexing entry note]: "Differential Diagnosis of Trigger Points." Gerwin, Robert. Co-published simultaneously in *Journal of Musculoskeletal Pain* [The Haworth Medical Press, an imprint of The Haworth Press, Inc.] Vol. 12, No. 3/4, 2004, pp. 23-28; and: *Soft Tissue Pain Syndromes: Clinical Diagnosis and Pathogenesis* [ed: Dieter E. Pongratz, Siegfried Mense, and Michael Spaeth] The Haworth Medical Press, an imprint of The Haworth Press, Inc., 2004, pp. 23-28. Single or multiple copies of this article are available for a fee from The Haworth Document Delivery Service [1-800-HAWORTH, 9:00 a.m. - 5:00 p.m. [EST]. E-mail address: docdelivery@haworthpress.com].

Available online at http://www.haworthpress.com/web/JMP
doi:10.1300/J094v12n03_04

pain syndromes. Ergonomic stresses include unaccustomed eccentric exercise or maximal exercise, as well as repetitive exercise syndromes.

Delayed onset muscle soreness is well known to occur after eccentric exercise, but has been shown to occur as well after ischemic exercise (1). Exercise under these conditions causes injury to the muscle fiber, and consequent pain or soreness. Muscle that is maximally eccentrically contracted shows evidence of muscle fiber destruction similar to changes seen in exercised ischemic muscle (2-4). Unaccustomed eccentric exercise also produces immediate damage to muscle and delayed muscle soreness in the succeeding days. Muscle soreness is the result of local muscle damage, inflammatory changes, and nociceptor sensitization (5). Repetitive exercise may entail repeated eccentric or lengthening contractions. A common example of this is keyboard entry, an activity that sometimes produces forearm pain and lateral epicondylalgia ["tennis elbow" or "gelato elbow"]. The source of injury in lateral epicondylalgia occurs during the "down-stroke" or lengthening phase of movement. For example, in making a keyboard stroke, the finger is flexed while the wrist remains held in an extended position, such that the extensor digitorum may be lengthened while contracted.

Hypermobility syndromes. These syndromes produce multiple mechanical stresses. Structural stress occurs as ligamentous laxity results in poor joint stabilization, muscles then being recruited to maintain joint integrity. This can result in a seemingly disproportionate number of hypermobile persons, mostly women, who have focal or generalized myalgia. In our experience, the affected muscles always have myofascial TrPs. Occasionally, there is full-blown Ehlers-Danlos syndrome with repeated shoulder or elbow dislocations. The mechanism of injury appears to be muscular stress or overload that arises from the effort required to maintain joint integrity. The most effective treatment is strengthening. In those women who have done this, shoulder dislocations and muscle pain have both ceased, and the women have been able to resume full activity, including sports activities, without further trouble.

Forward head posture places stress on the extensor muscles of the neck and shoulder [longissimus cervicis, semispinalis capitis and cervicis, splenius capitis and cervicis, the suboccipital muscles at the base of the skull, and the trapezius and levator scapulae muscles]. Forward head posture is often associated with posterior displacement of the mandible and temporomandibular joint pain. Posterior cervical muscle and shoulder muscle myalgic syndromes are thus frequently associated with head pain and headache.

Conversely, persons with myalgic headache often have mechanically induced myalgias. Myalgic headache is often the result of postural or ergonomic stress on the shoulder and neck muscles. Forward head posture certainly is seen in the older person with kypho-scoliosis, but can also be seen in young persons as well. Mouth-breathers are particularly susceptible to this. There is obstruction of the upper airway, the tongue is kept on the floor of the mouth to eliminate negative pressure with the palate, allowing the inferior airway to open. Bringing the head forward on the cervical spine facilitates opening the inferior airway. Consequently, the head-neck-shoulder relationships are altered, changing to a forward head posture (6). Children who present with headache, forward head posture, and muscle pain, need to be evaluated for allergies and other causes of upper airway obstruction.

Pelvic torsion-related pain is associated with pseudo-leg-length-inequality or with TrP muscular shortening [pseudoscoliosis]. It can be caused by, and in turn either cause or aggravate myalgia in lumbar muscles and in the pelvic floor muscles. Pelvic torsion causes an ipsilateral high posterior superior Iliac spine and a low anterior superior Iliac spine, indicating rotation of the pelvic iliac bone rather than leg length inequality. Treatment is derotation of the iliac bone. Muscle energy techniques are used to perform this corrective pelvic movement. Chronic muscle overload causes the pain. Scoliosis that results from pelvic torsion produces an asymmetry in shoulder height and a mechanical stress on neck and shoulders, which can cause myalgic headache, neck and shoulder pain. Hence, persons with headache, neck, and shoulder pain have their spine and pelvis evaluated for scoliosis and pelvic tilt and torsion.

Sacroiliac joint dysfunction. Sacroiliac joint dysfunction, or sacro-iliac joint hypomobility can cause pelvic and spine dysfunction that results in painful widespread axial muscle trigger points. Pain may be felt in the sacroiliac joint region [on either the hypomobile or the normal side], referred to the low back, or occur because of the secondary development of paraspinal TrP up the axial spine to the shoulders and neck.

Somatic dysfunction. Somatic dysfunction, or muscle-joint dysfunction, is a limitation of range of motion caused by a muscular restriction of joint motion. There may also be a persistent displacement of the bony part, expressed, for example, as a vertebral rotation or sideways displacement. These restrictions can be painful. They can be associated with palpable muscle TrPs or their persistence, and therefore are considered a cause of myalgia.

Static overload occurs when mechanically stressful positions are held for prolonged periods of time. This causes fatigue of the active muscles. Many conditions and habits can cause this, and it is a common workplace problem. The requirement to hold a fixed posture to, or past, muscle fatigue is the usual cause. Cradling the telephone between the ear and the shoulder creates scalene and trapezius muscle overload. This is much less common now, as it is such a well-known cause of neck and shoulder pain. Much less well known is mixed eye-hand dominance where the individual rotates the head to bring the dominant eye closer to reading material that is on the contralateral hand-dominant side. There are many variations of this, including the child-on-one-hip carry, seldom complained about, perhaps because mothers frequently expect to have backache when they have small children.

Nerve root compression can present with acute or chronic myofascial TrPs. Trigger point pain syndromes can develop acutely when there is an acute disc herniation. Muscle pain is in the distribution of the affected nerve root. It can precede any neurologic impairment such as weakness, sensory loss, paraesthesia, or reflex loss. Transient relief of the acute pain occurs with TrP therapy. Trigger point injection or needling can produce dramatic effects, but they last for only hours or days. Neurologic impairment always occurs within days of the onset of muscle pain, and is always severe. The TrPs recur acutely until the nerve root is decompressed. In every such case that we have seen, pain was severe and neurologic impairment progressed so rapidly that early surgery was always performed. We have also seen one case of T11 thoracic spinal cord ependymoma that presented in a similar manner, with the pain and TrP symptoms in the L1-2 dermatome distribution.

Muscle imbalance. Conditions in which muscle weakness causes an imbalance leading to mechanical asymmetries is often associated with MPSs. For example, 50 percent of persons with post-polio syndrome had symptomatic myofascial pain. In many cases, it was simply a matter of a leg-length inequality syndrome and low back pain, corrected by a heel lift and a butt lift to level the pelvis standing and sitting. For some reason, pain from similar structural adaptations to weakness is seen less often in our pain clinic in persons with hereditary myopathies. It is not clear if they do not have pain, or if they are simply told to expect pain and that there is no effective treatment for it.

The second major category is *Systemic medical illness*. The relationship of some of these conditions to myalgia has been difficult to confirm. Yet when such an illness is identified and treated, and muscle pain improves or resolves, it is tempting to equate the treatment with successful outcome. Nonetheless, one must be cautious about assuming a causal relationship. The conditions of interest include autoimmune disorders, infectious diseases, allergies, hormonal and nutritional deficiencies, viscerosomatic pain syndromes, and iatrogenic drug induced myalgic pain syndromes.

Autoimmune disorders. Muscle pain is a common accompanying symptom of many autoimmune disorders, particularly connective tissue diseases like lupus and Sjogren's syndrome. Polymyalgia rheumatica must certainly be considered in any head, neck, and shoulder regional muscular pain syndrome in an older [> 50 years of age] individual. Chewing-induced pain is an important component of both polymyalgia rheumatica and MPS, the latter when the temporomandibular joint is involved. Muscle pain may precede other signs of Sjogren's syndrome by several years. Physicians must be alert to the development of other signs, including sicca and xerostomia, and be willing to retest the patient over time.

Infectious diseases. Lyme disease is perhaps the most prevalent of the infectious diseases associated with myofascial pain. It is not known if there is a statistically significant association between these two conditions, but some persons with intractable widespread myalgia and chronic fatigue have been positive at significant titers for Lyme disease [IgG titers elevated, IgM titers normal, indicative of past, not recent, exposure]. Some of these patients also had arthralgia. Improvement occurred with doxycycline or azithromycin treatment for Lyme disease. Post-Lyme disease syndrome is characterized by diffuse arthralgia, myalgia, fatigue, and subjective cognitive difficulty (7). Patients diagnosed with this condition do not show evidence of chronic Borrelial infection, and they do not respond to a three-month course of antibiotics any better than a control group treated with placebo. There are also infectious disorders that present as chronic infections that look like Lyme disease, and that may co-infect with Lyme disease. These are Babesiosis, Ehrlichiosis, and Bartonella. Other infectious diseases of interest are *Mycoplasma* pneumonia and *Chlamydia* pneumonia. Interest in these two diseases arises because of a putative association with arthralgia or synovitis, in addition to an association with chronic fatigue and myalgia. The relationship is uncertain because of the widespread nature of these infections, many being asymptomatic. The outcome of long-term treatment of mycoplasma and chlamydia has been mixed. These two conditions are rather common, and serologic cross-reactivity may give false positive results. Any one of these infections, though there may be evidence of past contact, may be unrelated to myalgia, representing background noise or a non-specific anti-inflammatory response. Nevertheless, reduction of muscle discomfort with antibiotic treatment is clear in Lyme Disease. It is less clear in the cases *Mycoplasma* pneumonia and *Chlamydia* pneumonia.

We have also seen a number of patients with widespread myalgia and parasitic disease. The most common parasitic infections are amoebiasis and giardia. There is a single case of liver fluke infestation. Treatment of these conditions has generally resulted in a lessening or clearing of myalgia. Treatment of the patient with the liver fluke infestation resulted in complete resolution of myalgia. Treatment of the parasitic infection reduces or eliminates muscle pain.

Allergies. Cases of widespread myalgia [MPS] have been associated with persons who have had untreated allergies. Treatment of allergies has resulted in reduction or resolution of myalgia. The numbers involved are small. When the myalgic syndrome is limited to the head, neck and shoulders, forward head posture as described above, related to obstruction of the nasal passages, may play a role.

Viscero-somatic pain syndromes. Internal organs are associated with somatic segmental referred pain syndromes. Endometriosis, for example, is associated with abdominal myofascial pain (8). Interstitial cystitis and irritable bowel syndrome are associated with chronic pelvic pain syndromes (9-12). Liver disease can cause local abdominal and referred shoulder MPS that presents as a regional pain syndrome responsive to treatment of the TrPs by needling or by manual therapy.

Brain tumor and base of skull pain. Posterior fossa mass lesions [primary and metastatic tumors] can present as focal base of skull or upper cervical pain with identifiable myofascial TrPs that transiently respond to TrP inactivation.

NUTRITIONAL DEFICIENCIES

Vitamin D deficiency. One hundred and fifty consecutive patients between the ages of 15-65 years, attending clinic because of chronic nonspecific musculoskeletal pain were studied by Plotnikoff et al. (13). Exclusions included the diagnosis of FMS, temporomandibular joint dysfunction, and complex regional pain syndrome. Radioimmunoassay was used to determine the level of 25-OH vD. Normal vitamin D levels were > 20 ng/ml. Five-eight was severe deficiency and four or less was considered profound deficiency. The mean serum vitamin D levels in this group were 12 ng/ml. Eighty-nine percent of the persons in this group of chronic musculoskeletal pain were found to be deficient. This is an astounding figure that indicates that vitamin D deficiency is extremely common among those in the musculoskeletal pain community. The younger persons had lower serum vitamin D levels than the older population in the study.

Iron deficiency. Iron deficiency causes a metabolic stress that produces fatigue and muscle pain. We have been unable to document this (14,15), but treatment with iron supplements in women whose serum ferritin level is 20 pg/ml or less results in less fatigue, less coldness, and less muscle pain. We did not find a greater incidence of low serum ferritin levels in persons with MPS than without, despite our clinical impression that treatment with iron supplementation results in clinical improvement.

Iron insufficiency is also associated with restless leg syndrome, a cause of sleep disturbance. As noted above, sleep deprivation is a cause of myalgia. Thus, iron deficiency can aggravate muscle pain secondarily by causing restless leg syndrome.

DRUG INDUCED MYALGIA

Drugs can also cause muscle pain. Generally speaking, drug induced pain is widespread and diffuse, rather than regional. Drug-induced myalgia may or may not be associated with TrPs. Elevation of creatine kinase [CK] is a marker of muscle tissue breakdown, and is clearly a marker of an adverse muscle effect. However, CK is not necessarily elevated when there is drug-induced myalgia. Drugs known to produce myalgia, regardless of whether or not CK is elevated, include propoxyphene, and the statin family of cholesterol lowering drugs (16). The risk of acquiring myalgia is increased when a statin-drug is taken concomitantly with fibric acid derivative like gemfibrozil, niacin, Cyclosporine, Azole-antifungal and macrolide antibiotics, protease inhibitors, Nefazadone, verapamil, diltiazem, amiodarone, and grapefruit juice [> 1 qt/day].

CONCLUSION

Muscle pain can be the result of a wide-array of clinical conditions. In this review, I have not mentioned the inflammatory diseases of muscle such as polymyositis, or the inherited myopathies, although they, too, can present with pain. Myoadenylate deaminase deficiency is the most common inherited muscle enzyme disorder, but the role that it plays in muscle pain is still no clearer today than it was 10 years ago. Nevertheless, there are a number of conditions that can produce muscle pain that must be identified and addressed if patients are to recover.

REFERENCES

1. Barlas P, Walsh DM, Baxter GD, Allen JM. Delayed onset muscle soreness: Effect of an ischemic block upon mechanical allodynia in humans. Pain 87:221-225, 2000.

2. Crenshaw AG, Thornell LE, Friden J. Intramuscular pressure, torque and swelling for the exercise induced sore vastus lateralis muscle. Acta Physiol Scand 152:265-277, 1994.

3. Stauber WT, Clarkson DM, Fritz VK, Evans WJ. Extracellular matrix disruption and pain after eccentric muscle action. J Applied Physiol 69:868-874, 2002.

4. Trappe TA, Carrithers JA, White F, Lambert CP, Evans WJ, Dennis RA. Titin and nebulin content in human skeletal muscle following eccentric resistance exercise. Muscle Nerve 25:289-292, 2002.

5. Proske V, Morgan DC. Muscle damage from eccentric exercise: Mechanism, mechanical signs, adaptation and clinical applications. J Physiol 537:333-345, 2001.

6. Rocabado M, Iglarsh AZ. Musculoskeletal Approach to Maxillofacial Pain. Lippincott, Philadelphia, 1991, pp. 136-137.

7. Weinstein A, Britchkov M. Lyme arthritis and post-Lyme disease syndrome. Current Opinion in Rheumatology 14:383-387, 2002.

8. Jarrell J, Robert M. Myofascial dysfunction and pelvic pain. The Canadian J of CME Feb: 107-116, 2003

9. Weiss JM. Pelvic floor myofascial trigger points: Manual therapy for interstitial cystitis and the urgency-frequency syndrome. The Journal of Urology 166: 2226-2231, 2001.

10. Wiygul RD, Wiygul JP. Interstitial cystitis, pelvic pain, and the relationship to myofascial pain and dysfunction: A report on four patients. World J Urol 20:310-314, 2002.

11. Hetrick DC, Ciol MA, Rothman I, Turner JA, Frest M, Berger RE. Musculoskeletal dysfunction in men with chronic pelvic pain syndrome type III: A case-control study. J Urology 170:828-831, 2003.

12. Zermann DH, Ishigooka M, Doggweiler R, Schmidt RA. Chronic prostatitis: A myofascial pain syndrome? Urol 12:84-92, 1999.

13. Plotnikoff GA, Quigley JM. Prevalence of severe hypovitaminosis D in patients with persistent, nonspecific musculoskeletal pain. Mayo Clin Proc 78:1463-1470, 2003.

14. Gerwin RD, Gambel J, Shannon S, Rubertone M. A comparison of two possible perpetuating factors in a

military and a civilian population. J Musculoskel Pain 9 (Suppl 5):83 (Abs), 2001.

15. Gambel J, Shannon S, Rubertone M, Howard R, Gerwin R. Comparison of biochemical markers between active duty U.S. service members with chronic myo-

fascial pain and matched controls. J Musculoskel Pain 9 (Suppl 5): 85 (Abs), 2001.

16. Thompson PD, Clarkson P, Karas RH. Statin-associated myopathy. JAMA 289:1681-1690, 2003.

Trigger Points as a Cause of Orofacial Pain

Sandro Palla

SUMMARY. Orofacial pain is a common symptom experienced by approximately one-quarter of the adult population and is most often caused by myofascial pain. In contrast to other postural body muscles, trigger points are not often found in the jaw elevator muscles. Therefore, the term myofascial pain used in this article refers to a muscle pain condition characterized by the presence of muscle tenderness.

The masticatory myofascial pain, that may be triggered by oral parafunction during the awake state, often fluctuates with pain episodes followed by pain-free intervals. Especially non-chronic light to mild masticatory myofascial pain often resolves spontaneously. In each case non-chronic pain can be easily treated by a therapeutic plan that includes patient education, self-care, physiotherapy, pharmacotherapy, and eventually an occlusal appliance. Only in a small percent of patients does the masticatory myofascial pain become chronic. These patients need a multimodal therapeutic approach that addresses both the somatic and non-somatic, i.e., the emotional, affective, and behavioral pain component. Tricyclic antidepressants can be prescribed for the treatment of the somatic component while the therapy of the non-somatic component requires a cognitive-behavioral therapy. *[Article copies available for a fee from The Haworth Document Delivery Service: 1-800-HAWORTH. E-mail address: <docdelivery@haworthpress.com> Website: <http://www.HaworthPress. com> © 2004 by The Haworth Press, Inc. All rights reserved.]*

KEYWORDS. Myofascial pain, orofacial pain, masticatory myofascial pain

Orofacial pain is a common symptom experienced by approximately one-quarter of the adult population, of whom only one half seeks treatment. The prevalence is higher in women and younger age groups (1). The causes are numerous and may encompass pathologies in various tissues [pulpal, parodontal, articular, muscular] or organs [sinus, ears, eyes, intracranial structures]. Orofacial pain can also be an ectopic headache manifestation. Persistent orofacial pain is, however, most often due to myofascial pain.

The term myofascial pain is used in the literature with a general and a specific meaning. The specific meaning relates to a pain condition caused by myofascial trigger points [TrPs] while the general meaning indicates a regional muscle pain syndrome that is associated with muscle tenderness (2). Tender points are different from TrPs as they only elicit a localized pain at the site of palpation and not the referred pain that is one of the clinical characteristics of TrPs. The others include: 1. circumscribed spot tenderness in a small nodule situated within a palpable taut band, 2. recognition of the pain that is evoked by pressure on the nodule as being familiar [only in case of an active TrP], 3. local twitch response [LTR] upon stimulation of the

Sandro Palla, Prof. Dr., is affiliated with the Clinic for Masticatory Disorders and Complete Dentures, University of Zurich, CH-8028 Zurich, Switzerland [E-mail: palla@zzmk.unizh.ch].

[Haworth co-indexing entry note]: "Trigger Points as a Cause of Orofacial Pain." Palla, Sandro. Co-published simultaneously in *Journal of Musculoskeletal Pain* [The Haworth Medical Press, an imprint of The Haworth Press, Inc.] Vol. 12, No. 3/4, 2004, pp. 29-36; and: *Soft Tissue Pain Syndromes: Clinical Diagnosis and Pathogenesis* [ed: Dieter E. Pongratz, Siegfried Mense, and Michael Spaeth] The Haworth Medical Press, an imprint of The Haworth Press, Inc., 2004, pp. 29-36. Single or multiple copies of this article are available for a fee from The Haworth Document Delivery Service [1-800-HAWORTH, 9:00 a.m. - 5:00 p.m. [EST]. E-mail address: docdelivery@haworthpress.com].

Available online at http://www.haworthpress.com/web/JMP
© 2004 by The Haworth Press, Inc. All rights reserved.
doi:10.1300/J094v12n03_05

TrP, 4. painful limitation of muscle stretching, and 5. muscle weakness (3). Clinically TrPs are diagnosed by the presence of an hyperritable, hyperalgesic spot within a taut band that produces referred pain on compression. When this elicits the same pain usually felt by the patient, the TrP is active.

Thus, the type of pain referral differentiates an active from a latent TrP. This does not elicit pain at rest, is not responsible for the patient's pain, and elicits pain or discomfort only on compression. Only active TrPs produce clinical symptoms and usually produce more pronounced examination findings (2-4). Furthermore, dry needling of a latent TrP elicits the LTR only in the muscle with the TrP while needling of an active TrP evokes a LTR, in both the muscle with the TrP as well as in the contralateral one. This observation led the authors to hypothesize a loss of central inhibition of the contralateral reflex in the presence of active TrPs due to an abnormal processing of the noxious inputs into the central nervous system, i.e., to the neuroplastic changes caused by the incoming nociceptive barrage (5).

TRIGGER POINTS AND OROFACIAL PAIN

It has been reported that latent TrPs are common in a general population and that they may become active, i.e., painful at one given time or another (2). It is, however, not known if latent TrPs are frequently found also in masticatory muscles, as most clinical and epidemiological studies reported solely the prevalence of masticatory muscle tenderness to palpation and not of TrPs or of taut bands. Masticatory muscle tenderness is, nevertheless, also a common finding in a general population (6,7).

There are a few reports indicating that TrPs in the masticatory, neck, and shoulder muscles, diagnosed when palpation resulted in referred pain similar to that experienced by the patient, cause orofacial pain, toothache, and headache (8-11). For instance, specific areas of orofacial pain were consistently found to be associated with TrPs in masticatory, neck, and shoulder muscles in a group of patients with complaints of facial, head, and neck pain of more than six months duration. Temporomandibular joint pain

was elicited by TrPs in the deep masseter, middle and deep part of the temporal muscle, medial and lateral pterygoid muscle, and digastric muscle while jaw pain by TrPs in the superficial masseter, pterygoid, digastric, and trapezius muscle. This is probably the most comprehensive study on TrPs and orofacial pain (8). However, as several TrPs were located in muscles not accessible to palpation its value is limited to the TrPs found in the masseter and temporal muscle, the only palpable masticatory muscles.

Because of the lack of knowledge on the presence of TrPs in masticatory muscles and the author's clinical experience that TrPs are seldom present in these muscles, the following remarks consider myofascial pain as a regional muscle pain syndrome associated with muscle tenderness but not necessarily with TrPs.

MASTICATORY MYOFASCIAL PAIN

The etiology and the pathophysiologic mechanisms of masticatory myofascial pain [MMP] are so far poorly understood. According to the prevailing multifactorial etiologic concept, many predisposing, initiating, and perpetuating factors are involved. Risk factors that are always discussed in the literature are: occlusal parafunction [tooth clenching or grinding], gender, age, depression, and psychological and emotional trauma (12,13).

Episodic or acute MMP is likely precipitated by muscle fiber lesions caused by muscle overload or by repeated overuse. In 1991 Hägg postulated the cinderella hypothesis that states that during low-level contractions specific motor units [MUs] may be continuously active so that they become overloaded (14). The hypothesis is still not fully validated, though continuously active MUs have been found in the trapezius muscle while subjects were working with a computer mouse during a 30-minute period (15).

The mandible is supported against gravity in its habitual, postural position by a low degree of tonic contraction of the elevator muscles: the teeth are slightly apart (16). The clinical experience shows, however, that many patients with myofascial pain do not keep the masticatory muscles relaxed but have the tendency to keep the teeth in contact or to clench when awake and preliminary data indicates that patients with myofascial pain do in fact keep more often the teeth in contact than normal subjects [unpublished data]. This "unintentional" muscle tension,[1] that in dentistry is called parafunctional muscle activity, may be accompanied by continuously active MUs leading to muscle fibers overuse and therefore to TrPs. In this context it is important to point out two facts:

1. Motor-unit territories in the human masseter are focally distributed with a preferred orientation in the antero-posterior direction and are related to anatomical compartments (18). The restriction of these territories to discrete regions of the muscle provides an anatomical substrate for selective regional motor control of the masseter muscle. As a consequence it is possible that during parafunctional activity selected muscle areas are contracted for longer period of time leading to muscle fiber lesions and therefore to pain through muscle nociceptors sensitization.

2. A causal relationship between bruxism and MMP is often denied in the literature because only a small minority of sleep bruxers awake with orofacial pain. However, most epidemiological studies reported a significant though low association between oral habits/occlusal parafunction and myofascial pain. The fact that this association is generally low does not surprise, being that the etiology is multicausal. Nevertheless, it is likely that sleep bruxism represents a lower risk factor for MMP than non-sleep parafunction because this reproduces more the conditions of a long-lasting muscle contraction or of a repetitive overuse.

DIAGNOSIS OF MASTICATORY MYOFASCIAL PAIN

The diagnosis of a myofascial pain relies on a thorough pain history and a clinical examination. In absence of laboratory or other specific tests muscle palpation and functional testing remain the essential element of diagnostic significance. A MMP is diagnosed when, in presence of facial, auricular, preauricular, temporal or jaw pain at rest or during jaw function, at least three out of 14 muscle areas are tender to palpation. One of the tender spots must be located on the painful side. The muscle sites to be palpated are the superficial and deep masseter, the anterior, middle and posterior part of the temporal muscle as well as the insertions of the temporal and medial pterygoid muscles. The examination of the cervical spine and their soft tissues is mandatory in patients with orofacial pain because cervical, neck, and paraspinal muscles refer the pain also to the head and orofacial area as it has been documented by the intramuscular injection of algesic substances as well as in case reports (8,9,19-21).

The presence of muscle tenderness does not warrant per se a diagnosis of myofascial pain. Indeed, tenderness to palpation has a low sensitivity, a somewhat higher specificity, and a very low positive predictive value (22). There are several factors that contribute to these low values. First, tender areas on palpation are also found in normal individuals free of orofacial, head, and shoulder-neck pain but are less frequent and less tender than in patients (6). Second, palpation tenderness is very technique sensitive (23). Third, studies on pain pressure threshold indicate that a local tenderness must not be related to a local pathology. Indeed, the pain pressure threshold is not any lower on the painful than on the non-painful side (24) and, what is even more important, normal individuals have a higher threshold than patients with fibromyalgia, myofascial pain, or a non-myogeneous pain (24-27). In addition, in these patients the pressure pain threshold is lower also at placebo sites, i.e., on anatomical sides free of muscles (27). These observations indicate that increased tenderness may simply reflect increased pain sensitivity, i.e., secondary hyperalgesia. This is not caused by peripheral nociceptor sensitization but by central sensitization of the second order neurons (2). Thus, the main diagnostic question to be answered when evaluating muscle tenderness to palpation is whether this reflects primary or secondary hyperalgesia because only a primary hyperalgesia warrants the diagnosis of a MMP.

Also the presence of a taut band is not per se a sign of a muscle disorder as taut bands are found also in pain-free subjects without other clinical evidence of TrPs phenomena (28).

As pain in general also the MMP is experienced by patients in an individual manner and may lead to behaviors that are detrimental for his/her life as well as that of his/her family. While in non-chronic pain patients the accent in the diagnostic process is on the organic diagnosis, in chronic pain patients it is mandatory to evaluate the implications that the pain has on daily living, i.e., the global severity of the pain condition in terms of pain intensity, pain-related disability, depression, somatization as well as the consequences that the pain condition has on the behavioral and emotional status of the patient. Indeed, in terms of levels of pain intensity and interference and psychologic and psychosocial profiles, chronic MMP is similar to many other common pain problems, such as low back pain and headache (29). Psychologic factors are also seen as the most important risk factors for chronicity (30-33). This is important as the chronic pain patient needs a multidisciplinary therapy that also addresses the non-somatic aspects of the pain.

As a consequence, the diagnostic process differs if we are dealing with a non-chronic or a chronic MMP. For chronic pain patients it is mandatory to make both a somatic and a psychosocial diagnosis in order to understand how biomedical and psychosocial factors interact to determine the severity and persistence of the pain condition.

THERAPY

The following principles for the management of myofascial pain reflect the evidence from the literature, and the clinical author's experience. They are based on the hypothesis that muscle overuse plays an important role in the etiology of the episodic pain, while central hyperexcitability, neuronal plasticity and/or a dysregulation of the descending nociceptive system as well as a dysfunctional pain adaptation model with all its psychosocial implications are involved in patients with persistent, chronic MMP, that, however, develops in a minority of cases, usually less than 20 percent.

The therapy should be divided into:

- Therapy of non-chronic forms
- Management of chronic forms

In the therapeutic context the difference between acute and chronic pain does not primarily refer to the pain duration [> three or six months] but on the presence or absence of somatosensoric disturbances and of accompanying affective, emotional, and behavioral features, i.e., of behavioral and existential orientation disturbances. Therefore, therapy of myofascial pain is based on an individualized multimodal and interdisciplinary approach that depends on the dimension of disability and degree of the chronification process.

Non-Chronic Form

Treatment goals for patients with MMP include pain alleviation, decreased loading of the masticatory muscles, and restored oral function. Though well designed prospective and/or randomized clinical studies that use appropriate outcome measures and controls to validate the results of MMP therapy are just starting to appear, it seems safe to state that non-chronic forms can be safely and effectively treated by means of a simple therapeutic program that includes patient education and self-care, physical therapy, pharmacotherapy, and eventually an occlusal appliance.

In any case, treatment must begin with the patient having correct information. Inform the patient of the diagnosis, the presumed etiology, assure the patient that there is no dangerous problem and that muscle pain is often self-limiting and resolves without apparent side effects. The patient with MMP must learn to avoid occlusal or oral parafunctional activity, to keep the muscle relaxed by holding the mandible in its postural position and not in occlusion, as this jaw position requires "unintentional" muscle tension, and to learn a correct head position. Another goal of counseling is to motivate the patient to recognize if he/she performs oral habits and to identify the factors or the situations that may trigger them. Considering that patients with myofascial pain may display a deficit in the discrimination of muscle tension (34) and that proprioceptive awareness may vary as a function of situational stress (35), it is tenable to suppose that these patients may use high levels of muscle tension when keeping the teeth in contact without awareness.

Physiotherapy. The aim includes restoration of the muscle to its normal length, posture, and full range of motion. In our experience a short home physiotherapy program that includes application of cold/hot packs [two times for 20 minutes], self-massage, stretching exercises [6 × 6 × a day for six seconds every stretch], exercises for head posture and eventually also co-ordination and stabilization exercises should be prescribed to every patient. Patients with concomitant myofascial pain in the neck and/or shoulder area should be referred to a physical therapist for specific treatment.

Though the true efficacy of such a program has never been proved in randomized clinical trials, patients with MMP should be instructed from the beginning in the home program. Indeed, the combination of counseling and home program seems to provide a better subjective improvement than the other two single therapies. The better success of the combination treatment group was, however, related not to the physiotherapy but to the fact that patients who received the home program felt they received a better therapy than those who received only counseling (36).

Despite lack of evidence, the proposed home program has the great advantage to involve the patient from the beginning in the management of his/her pain condition and to make him/her feel responsible for the recovery.

Pharmacologic treatment. There is little evidence of efficacy of pharmacotherapy in MMP as reported in two recent literature reviews on randomized controlled studies (37,38). Nonsteroidal anti-inflammatory drugs are certainly contraindicated as they aim to reduce pain in inflamed conditions which is not the case for myofascial pain and indeed nonsteroidal anti-inflammatory drugs are ineffective for MMP (39). There is, however, at least a low degree of evidence for the use of muscle relaxants as an adjunctive therapy (39,40). A randomized controlled study reported that a centrally acting muscle relaxant [cyclobenzaprine] given one hour before bedtime was more effective than clonazepam or placebo for patients with orofacial pain on awakening (40). Another centrally acting muscle relaxant, that according to

an open label trial is effective in the therapy of MMP, is Tizanidin.

Relaxation therapy. Autogenous training, progressive muscle relaxation and biofeedback are often effectively used to treat MMP. For instance, biofeedback, the relaxation therapy most often used and investigated, is effective in relieving MMP (41). Its mechanism of action is, however, not specific as the therapeutic effect occurs independently of a reduction of the muscle tone and is likely behavioral in nature (41,42). Biofeedback is very helpful to teach patients how to relax the elevator muscles so that they can learn to keep the mandible in the postural position.

Occlusal appliances. A therapy form specifically used to treat MMP are occlusal appliances. Their effectiveness in alleviating pain is well documented in several case series: pain remission or alleviation is reached in 70-80 percent of the patients. One of two recently published systematic literature reviews (43,44) conclude that, though the efficacy of occlusal appliances is not proven, the results of the latest randomized control studies (45-47) may give support to their use (44). The other review reported that there is weak evidence suggesting that the use of occlusal appliances may be beneficial for reducing pain severity, at rest and on palpation, when compared to no treatment (43). Because of this lack of evidence, occlusal appliances should not be the first treatment modality but should be prescribed when the previously described therapies are not effective [Figure 1]. An exception are those patients who wake up with MMP because an oral splint may reduce sleep bruxism (48).

FIGURE 1. Flow chart diagram of the therapy of a non-chronic masticatory myofascial pain.

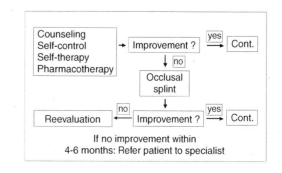

The occlusal appliances mechanism of action is still poorly understood and this is reflected by the fact that even occlusal appliances with completely different occlusal designs are in general almost equally effective. Recent data showing that the insertion of an occlusal appliance leads to a shift in the antero-posterior recruitment pattern of motor units (49) may support the hypothesis that occlusal appliances work because the new recruitment pattern unloads the overused muscle fibers.

Trigger point needling. Trigger points are often treated by injection [wet needling] or dry needling which are equally effective (50) but there is a lack of literature on the effect TrPs injection on MMP and in our experience TrP injections are seldom needed to treat MMP. In any case the injections should be integrated into a multimodal therapeutic concept including physical therapy and relaxation exercises (51).

Management of Chronic Myalgia

The therapy of these pain conditions may be very difficult and the goal of pain remission can not always be achieved. Often only the goals of pain reduction and of a better coping with the pain can be reached. Therefore, it is important to discuss with the patient right from the beginning the therapeutic goals in order to avoid unrealistic expectations.

Chronic myofascial pain can not be treated like an acute condition. First, the neuroplastic changes require other drug classes than those used for the treatment of acute pain. Second, the non-somatic pain dimension must be treated too. Chronic pain patients react to the myalgic pain with the involvement of the entire personality.

Patients with chronic myofascial pain must be managed with a multimodal approach so that the different somatic, affective, emotional, and behavioral pain aspects as well as other co-morbid pain conditions, like headache, atypical facial pain, or fibromyalgia are treated simultaneously. The above mentioned therapies are integrated with cognitive-behavioral therapy and pharmacological interventions that may treat, if necessary, also mood and sleep disorders.

Cognitive-behavioral therapy. This therapy, that is an integral part of each management program for patients with chronic pain (52), acts on two levels: it helps the patient through the learn-

ing of new coping strategies to change his reaction type to pain triggering or pain increasing situations and to learn a positive coping attitude towards the pain. The feeling of helplessness and of lack of control are reduced so that the patient can better control the pain. He/she must learn that the affective, emotional pain component is as important as the somatic one. The primary goal of the cognitive-behavioral therapy is therefore not pain reduction but to learn a better pain coping strategy, i.e., a better quality of life in the presence of pain. Relaxation therapy is an important component of the cognitive-behavioral therapy as it reduces the pain induced tension, distracts from pain and provides a feeling of self-efficacy (53).

Pharmacological therapy. In the case of chronic MMP, tricyclic antidepressants, especially those with an adrenergic and serotoninergic action, are indicated. The analgesic action of the antidepressants is well documented. They are effective also in the treatment of MMP. Pain remission does not occur as rapidly as with the use of the analgesics and is often uncompleted: not all patients react in the same way. Antidepressants lead to side effects caused by their anticholinergic action. As the side effects occur especially at the beginning of the therapy, the dosage must be slowly increased until pain remission occurs or the patient no longer tolerates the side effects. The antidepressants of the new generation have less side effects but seem to be also less effective in their analgesic action. The sedative effect of several antidepressants can be used to improve the sleep that is often disturbed in chronic pain patients.

In conclusion, chronic persistent MMP must be treated with a multimodal approach in order to address simultaneously both the somatic and the non-somatic pain component. The cognitive-behavioral therapy is not an additional therapy but an integral component of the therapeutic plan, i.e., it must be integrated from the beginning and not after another failure of another somatic treatment approach.

NOTE

1. "Unnecessary" or "unintentional" muscle tension is a confusing intermediate between muscle contraction that is beyond voluntary control and viscoelastic tension

without EMG activity. The sources of this unintentional activity are psychological stress or anxiety, overload from sustained contraction or repetitive work and inefficient [untrained] use of muscle (17).

REFERENCES

1. Macfarlane TV, Blinkhorn AS, Davies RM, Kincey J, Worthington HV: Oro-facial pain in the community: prevalence and associated impact. Community Dent Oral Epidemiol 30: 52-60, 2002.

2. Mense S, Simons DG, Russell IJ: Muscle Pain. Understanding its nature, diagnosis, and treatment. Lippincott, Williams & Williams, Philadelphia, 2001, p. 205.

3. Simons DG: Review of enigmatic TrPs as a common cause of enigmatic musculoskeletal pain and dysfunction. J Electromyogr Kinesiol 14: 95-107, 2004.

4. Hong CZ, Chen YN, Twehous DA, Hong DA: Pressure threshold for referred pain by compression on the trigger point and adjacent areas. J Musculoskeletal Pain 4(3): 61-79, 1996.

5. Audette JF, Wang F, Smith H: Bilateral activation of motor unit potentials with unilateral needle stimulation of active myofascial trigger points. Am J Phys Med Rehabil 83: 368-374, 2004.

6. Dworkin SF, Huggins KH, LeResche L, Von Korff M, Howard J, Truelove E, Sommers E: Epidemiology of signs and symptoms in temporomandibular disorders: Clinical signs in cases and controls. J Am Dent Assoc 120: 273-281, 1990.

7. Gesch D, Bernhardt O, Alte D, Schwahn C, Kocher T, John U, Hensel E: Prevalence of signs and symptoms of temporomandibular disorders in an urban and rural German population: Results of a population-based Study of Health in Pomerania. Quintessence Int 35: 143-150, 2004.

8. Fricton JR, Kroening R, Haley D, Siegert R: Myofascial pain syndrome of the head and neck: A review of clinical characteristics of 164 patients. Oral Surg Oral Med Oral Pathol 60: 615-623, 1985.

9. Jaeger B: Are "cervicogenic" headaches due to myofascial pain and cervical spine dysfunction? Cephalalgia 9: 157-164, 1989.

10. Konzelman JL, Herman WW, Comer RW: Pseudo-dental pain and sensitivity to percussion. Gen Dent 49: 156-158, 2001.

11. Mascia P, Brown BR, Friedman S: Toothache of nonodontogenic origin: A case report. J Endod 29: 608-610, 2003.

12. LeResche L: Epidemiology of temporomandibular disorders: Implications for the investigation of etiologic factors. Crit Rev Oral Biol Med 8: 291-305, 1997.

13. Palla S: Myoarthropatischer Schmerz des Kausystems (Myoarthropatic pain of the masticatory system).Chronischer Muskelschmerz (Chronic muscle pain). Edited by S Mense, D Pongratz. Steinkopff, Darmstadt, p. 145, 2002.

14. Hägg GM: Static work and myalgia–A new explanation model. Electromyographical kinesiology. Edited by PA Andersson, GJ Hobart, JV Danoff. Elsevier Science, Amsterdam, pp. 115-199, 1991.

15. Zennaro D, Laubli T, Krebs D, Klipstein A, Krueger H: Continuous, intermitted and sporadic motor unit activity in the trapezius muscle during prolonged computer work. J Electromyogr Kinesiol 13: 113-124, 2003.

16. Woda A, Piochon P, Palla S: Regulation of mandibular postures: mechanisms and clinical implications. Crit Rev Oral Biol Med 12: 166-178, 2001.

17. Simons DG, Mense S: Understanding and measurement of muscle tone as related to clinical muscle pain. Pain 75: 1-17, 1998.

18. McMillan AS, Hannam AG: Motor-unit territory in the human masseter muscle. Arch Oral Biol. 36: 435-441, 1991.

19. Simons DG, Travell JG, Simons LS: Travell and Simons' Myofascial pain and dysfunction. The trigger point manual. Volume 1. Upper half of the body. 2 ed. Williams & Wilkins, Baltimore, 1999.

20. Carlson CR, Okeson JP, Falace DA, Nitz AJ, Lindroth JE: Reduction of pain and EMG activity in the masseter region by trapezius trigger point injection. Pain 55: 397-400, 1993.

21. Davidoff RA: Trigger points and myofascial pain: Toward understanding how they affect headaches. Cephalalgia 18: 436-448, 1998.

22. Widmer CG: Physical characteristics associated with temporomandibular disorders. Temporomandibular disorders and related pain conditions. Edited by BJ Sessle, PS Bryant, RA Dionne. IASP Press, Seattle, pp. 161-174, 1995.

23. Jensen K: Quantification of tenderness by palpation and use of pressure algometers. Edited by JR Fricton, EA Awad. Raven Press, New York, pp. 165-181, 1990.

24. Reid KI, Gracely RH, Dubner RA: The influence of time, facial side, and location on pain-pressure thresholds in chronic myogenous temporomandibular disorder. J Orofac Pain 8: 258-265, 1994.

25. McMillan AS, Blasberg B: Pain-pressure threshold in painful jaw muscles following trigger point injection. J Orofac Pain 8: 384-390, 1994.

26. Tunks E, Crook J, Norman G, Kalaher S: Tender points in fibromyalgia. Pain 34: 11-19, 1988.

27. Tunks E, McCain GA, Hart LE, Teasell RW, Goldsmith CH, Rollman GB, McDermid AJ, DeShane PJ: The reliability of examination for tenderness in patients with myofascial pain, chronic fibromyalgia and controls. J Rheumatol 22: 944-952, 1995.

28. Fricton JR: Myofascial pain: clinical characteristics and diagnostic criteria. J Musculoskeletal Pain 1 (3/4): 37-47, 1993.

29. Von Korff M, Ormel J, Keefe FJ, Dworkin SF: Grading the severity of chronic pain. Pain 50: 133-149, 1992.

30. Epker J, Gatchel RJ: Coping profile differences in the biopsychosocial functioning of patients with tem-

poromandibular disorder. Psychosom Med 62: 69-75, 2000.

31. Hasenbring M: Byopsychosoziale Grundlagen der Chronifizierung am Beispiel von Rückenschmerzen (Biopsychosocial basis of pain chronification explained on the basis of back pain). Lerhbuch der Schmerztherapie. Edited by M Zenz, I Jurna. Wissenschaftliche Verlagsgesellschaft, Stuttgart, pp. 185-196, 2001.

32. Linton SJ: Psychological risk factors as "yellow flags" for back pain. Pain 2002–An updated review: Refresher course Syllabus. Edited by MA Giamberardino. IASP Press, Seattle, pp. 271-277, 2002.

33. Turk DC: The role of demographic and psychosocial factors in transition from acute to chronic pain. Proceedings of the 8th world congress on pain. Edited by TS Jensen, JA Turner, Z Wiesenfeld-Hallin. IASP Press, Seattle, pp. 185-213, 1997.

34. Flor H, Schugens MM, Birbaumer N: Discrimination of muscle tension in chronic pain patients and healthy controls. Biofeedback Self Regul 17: 165-177, 1992.

35. Glaros AG: Awareness of physiological responding under stress and nonstress conditions in temporomandibular disorders. Biofeedback Self Regul 21: 261-272, 1996.

36. Michelotti A, Parisini F, Farella M, Cimino R, Martina R: [Muscular physiotherapy in patients with temporomandibular disorders. Controlled clinical trial]. Minerva Stomatol 49: 541-548, 2000.

37. List T, Axelsson S, Leijon G: Pharmacologic interventions in the treatment of temporomandibular disorders, atypical facial pain, and burning mouth syndrome. A qualitative systematic review. J Orofac Pain 17: 301-310, 2003.

38. Sommer C: Pharmakologische Behandlung orofazialer Schmerzen [Pharmacotherapy of orofacial pain]. Schmerz 16: 381-388, 2002.

39. Singer E, Dionne R: A Controlled Evaluation of Ibuprofen and Diazepam for Chronic Orofacial Muscle Pain. J Orofac Pain 11: 139-146, 1997.

40. Herman CR, Schiffman EL, Look JO, Rindal DB: The effectiveness of adding pharmacologic treatment with clonazepam or cyclobenzaprine to patient education and self-care for the treatment of jaw pain upon awakening: A randomized clinical trial. J Orofac Pain 16: 64-70, 2002.

41. Crider AB, Glaros AG: A meta-analysis of EMG biofeedback treatment of temporomandibular disorders. J Orofac Pain 13: 29-37, 1999.

42. Kröner-Herwig B: Biofeedback. Psychologische Schmerztherapie (Psycological pain therapy). Edited by

H-D Basler, C Franz, B Kröner-Herwig. Springer, Berlin, pp. 627-643, 1999.

43. Al Ani MZ, Davies SJ, Gray RJ, Sloan P, Glenny AM: Stabilisation splint therapy for temporomandibular pain dysfunction syndrome. Cochrane Database Syst Rev CD002778, 2004.

44. Forssell H, Kalso E: Application of principles of evidence-based medicine to occlusal treatment for temporomandibular disorders: Are there lessons to be learned? J Orofac Pain 18: 9-22, 2004.

45. Dao TT, Lund JP, Lavigne GJ: Comparison of pain and quality of life in bruxers and patients with myofascial pain of the masticatory muscles. J Orofac Pain 8: 350-356, 1994.

46. Ekberg E, Vallon D, Nilner M: The efficacy of appliance therapy in patients with temporomandibular disorders of mainly myogenous origin. A randomized, controlled, short-term trial. J Orofac Pain 17: 133-139, 2003.

47. Raphael KG, Marbach JJ: Widespread pain and the effectiveness of oral splints in myofascial face pain. J Am Dent Assoc 132: 305-316, 2001.

48. Clark GT, Beemsterboer PL, Solberg WK, Rugh JD: Nocturnal electromyographic evaluation of myofascial pain dysfunction in patients undergoing occlusal splint therapy. J Am Dent Assoc 99: 607-611, 1979.

49. Schindler HJ, Rong Q, Spiess WEL: Der Einfluss von Aufbissschienen auf das Rekrutierungsmuster des Musculus temporalis (The influence of occlusal splints on the recruitment pattern of the temporal muscle). Dtsch Zahnarztl. Z 55: 575-581, 2000.

50. Cummings TM, White AR: Needling therapies in the management of myofascial trigger point pain: A systematic review. Arch Phys Med Rehabil 82: 986-992, 2001.

51. Reilich P, Fheodoroff K, Kern U, Mense S, Seddigh S, Wissel J, Pongratz D: Consensus statement: Botulinum toxin in myofacial pain. J Neurol. 251 Suppl 1: I36-I38, 2004.

52. Morley S, Eccleston C, Williams A: Systematic review and meta-analysis of randomized controlled trials of cognitive behaviour therapy and behaviour therapy for chronic pain in adults, excluding headache. Pain 80: 1-13, 1999.

53. Flor H, Turk DC: Der kognitiv-verhaltenstherapeutische Ansatz und seine Auswirkungen (Cognitive-behavioral therapy and its consequences). Psychologische Schmerztherapie (Psychological pain therapy). Edited by HD Basler, C Franz, B Kröner-Herwig, HP Rehfisch, H Seemann. Springer Verlag, Berlin, pp. 501-517, 1990.

Myofascial Pain Therapy

Chang-Zern Hong

SUMMARY. Background: The most important strategy in myofascial pain syndrome therapy is to identify the etiological lesion that causes the activation of myofascial trigger points[s] and to treat the underlying pathology. If the underlying etiological lesion is not appropriately treated, the TrP can only be inactivated temporarily, and never completely.

Findings: Generally, active TrPs should be treated conservatively with non-invasive techniques such as physical therapy prior to the consideration of aggressive therapy with invasive techniques such as needling and injection. This principle should also be observed when treating the underlying etiological lesions. Conservative therapy, such as manual therapy combined with thermotherapy and electrotherapy, can usually inactivate painful TrPs. Other situations, however, might necessitate dry needling or TrP injection: 1. persistent pain or discomfort after complete elimination of the underlying pathological lesion responsible for TrP activation, 2. poor response to conservative therapy, 3. intolerable pain, 4. deep location of a TrP, rendering it inaccessible by conservative manual therapy, 5. inadequate time to accept the time-consuming conservative therapy, or 6. personal preference. When treating myofascial pain syndrome, it is also important to eliminate any perpetuating factors that may cause persistent chronic pain, and to provide adequate education and home programs to patients, so that recurrent or chronic pain can be avoided.

Conclusions: Myofascial pain should be appropriately treated to inactivate TrPs completely and to avoid recurrence permanently. *[Article copies available for a fee from The Haworth Document Delivery Service: 1-800-HAWORTH. E-mail address: <docdelivery@haworthpress.com> Website: <http://www.HaworthPress.com> © 2004 by The Haworth Press, Inc. All rights reserved.]*

KEYWORDS. Myofascial pain syndrome, management, etiology perpetuating factors, trigger points

INTRODUCTION

The existence of myofascial trigger point [TrP] has now been widely accepted based on the facts of clinical observation and basic science research (1-24). There are multiple active TrP loci in a TrP region. A TrP locus consists of two components: the *sensitive locus [local twitch response [LTR locus]]* and the *active locus [end plate noise [EPN locus]]* (5-7,9). Basic science studies have suggested that a sensitive locus is a sensitized nerve ending (8), while an active locus is a dysfunctional endplate with excessive acetylcholine leakage (9,17-22). The excessive acetylcholine leakage may cause focal contracture of muscle fibers in

Chang-Zern Hong, MD, is affiliated with the Department of Physical Therapy, Hungkuang University, Tai-Chung, Taiwan and the Department of Physical Medicine and Rehabilitation, University of California Irvine, Irvine, CA, USA.

Address correspondence to: Chang-Zern Hong, MD, Department of Physical Therapy, Hungkuang University, 34 Chung-Chie Road, Shalu, Taichung, Taiwan [E-mail: czhong88@ms49.hinet.net or: czhong@uci.edu or: czh@sunrise.hk.edu.tw].

[Haworth co-indexing entry note]: "Myofascial Pain Therapy." Hong. Chang-Zern. Co-published simultaneously in *Journal of Musculoskeletal Pain* [The Haworth Medical Press, an imprint of The Haworth Press, Inc.] Vol. 12, No. 3/4, 2004, pp. 37-43; and: *Soft Tissue Pain Syndromes: Clinical Diagnosis and Pathogenesis* [ed: Dieter E. Pongratz, Siegfried Mense, and Michael Spaeth] The Haworth Medical Press, an imprint of The Haworth Press, Inc., 2004, pp. 37-43. Single or multiple copies of this article are available for a fee from The Haworth Document Delivery Service [1-800-HAWORTH, 9:00 a.m. - 5:00 p.m. [EST]. E-mail address: docdelivery@haworthpress.com].

Available online at http://www.haworthpress.com/web/JMP
© 2004 by The Haworth Press, Inc. All rights reserved.
doi:10.1300/J094v12n03_06

the endplate region, and subsequently becomes a taut band (18). We can identify the tenderest spot, the *latent TrP* [tender, but not painful spontaneously], in almost every normal skeletal muscle. The latent TrP can be activated to become an *active TrPM* [painful spontaneously or in response to movement] secondary to a certain pathological lesion. After appropriate treatment of this lesion, the active TrP can be suppressed to be inactive. The TrP never disappears, but just converts from one form to the other. Myofascial pain syndrome is a pain phenomenon due to activation of latent TrPs as a consequence of a certain pathological condition such as chronic repetitive minor muscle strain, poor posture, systemic disease, or soft tissue lesion (3,5-7,9,25). The treatment of underlying pathology is the fundamental approach in the management of TrPs. Myofascial pain therapy has been comprehensively described (22-24, 26-28). In this review, the basic principles, rather than the methods, of myofascial pain therapy are discussed.

MECHANISM
OF MYOFASICAL PAIN THERAPY

Peripheral Mechanism of Myofascial Pain Therapy

Simons had established the "energy crisis theory" more than 20 years ago (23). He suggested that a vicious cycle of energy crisis may occur when the energy [and oxygen] requirement for the persistent muscle contraction of the taut band is increased under the situation of impaired local circulation as a consequence of sustained compression to the microvasculature by the tight muscle fibers. Local muscle fiber contracture [with microscopic evidence of contractions of individual muscle fibers in the endplate zone of taut band (22)] can induce release of serotonin, histamine, bradykinin, and prostaglandin, which stimulate local nociception (16). Therefore, one major goal of TrP therapy is to release the taut band by using various methods of therapy.

Central Mechanism of Myofascial Pain Therapy

Two important characteristics of TrPs are referred pain [ReP] and LTR (9,22-24). Strong evidence from basic science studies (13-15) indicate that ReP is a central sensitization phenomenon in the spinal cord. Both clinical (2) and animal (10,11) studies have indicated that LTR is mainly mediated via spinal cord reflex. Hong has hypothesized that a "myofascial trigger point circuit" [MTrP circuit] in the spinal cord is the major center to control the TrP phenomena (7). When a mechanical stimulation is applied on the peripheral nociceptors in the TrP region, the neural impulses are transmitted via the TrP circuit to the cerebral cortex to cause local pain. Stronger impulses from a high-pressure stimulation may also be transmitted from the correspondent TrP circuit to the other TrP circuits of other TrPs to elicit ReP (4,7), or may elicit an LTR via a polysynaptic spinal cord reflex (6,7,9). The TrP circuit may be modified by a strong peripheral stimulus [high pressure massage or needling] so that the sensitivity is reduced, and thus, to block any painful impulse into the higher centers. This may be one basic mechanism of pain control by certain types of myofascial pain therapy (7).

BASIC PRINCIPLE
OF MYOFASCIAL PAIN THERAPY

Identification and Treatment of Underlying Pathological Lesions

Soft tissue lesions are the most common causes to activate the TrPs (3,5-7,9,29). The underlying etiological soft tissue lesions may be identified based on a careful clinical assessment. If the muscles with active TrPs are distributed in a myotome-pattern of a certain root, they are very likely caused by or related to radiculopathy of such root (30). When the TrPs are identified in the muscles around a joint, they are very likely caused by or related to sprain, synovitis, or arthritis of that joint. If the symptoms of TrPs are increased when a muscle actively contracts again resistance, it is very likely that they are related to or caused by a tendon lesion or enthesopathy of that muscle. When a certain facet joint is compressed or stretched, the TrP symptoms may be increased if they are caused by or related to facet joint lesion of such level (31,32).

Inactivation of Active Myofascial Trigger Points

If the pain still persists after the underlying etiological lesion[s] is [are] appropriately treated, the residual active TrPs should be treated to have a complete relief of pain. In some cases, the etiological lesion is unable to be accurately identified or adequately treated, TrP therapy is still required to control the severe pain. In many situations, release of muscle tightness after inactivation of TrPs can improve the local circulation to facilitate the healing process of the underlying etiological lesion. Release of muscle tightness can also increase the range of motion, and subsequently, can improve the functional activity. The commonly used methods for TrP therapy [inactivation of TrPs] are listed in Table 1. To inactivate TrPs, the following principles should be seriously considered.

1. *Pain Recognition*: It is important to confirm that the TrPs to be treated are those causing the usual complaint or discomfort of the patient. Do not treat the wrong TrPs [latent].

2. *Identification of Key TrP*: When a TrP becomes very active [hyperirritable], other latent TrPs may also be activated to active TrPs [satellite or secondary TrPs] that are usually distributed in the referred zone of the key [primary] TrP. The key TrP is much more painful than the

TABLE 1. Methods to Treat Active Myofascial Trigger Points

A. Manual Therapy
 1. Stretching–Intermittent Cold and Stretch.
 2. Deep Pressure Soft Tissue Massage.
 3. Trigger Point Pressure Release [Modified Myotherapy].
 4 Ischemic Compression, Acupressure, Myotherapy, Shiatzu.
 5. Chiropractic Therapy: Manipulation and Mobilization.
 6. Voluntary Contraction and Release Methods:
    1. Contract-Relax; Muscle Energy Technique.
    2. Reciprocal Inhibition.
    3. Post-Isometric Relaxation [Lewit].
 7. Others.
B. Modality Application [Physical Medicine]
 1. Thermotherapy.
 2. Electrotherapy.
 3. Laser Therapy.
 4. Others.
C. Needling
 1. Traditional Acupuncture.
 2. Dry Needling [Gunn, Chu, Baldry].
 3. Myofascial trigger point injection [Travell, Simons, Hong] and Preinjection Block [Fischer].
D. Others–Therapeutic Exercise, Medication, Biofeedback, Hypnosis, etc.
E. Combinations

---

satellite ones. To identify the key TrP, one can ask the patient to point out the most painful ones. If the key TrP is compressed, referred pain can be elicited or intensified in the satellite TrPs. On the other hand, if one of the satellite TrPs is compressed, no referred pain to the key TrP can be elicited.

3. *Conservative versus Aggressive Therapy*: Active TrPs should be treated conservatively [non-invasive treatment including physical therapy] prior to the consideration of aggressive therapy [invasive treatment including injection and surgery]. This principle is similarly applied on the treatment of the underlying etiological lesions. Other situations, however, might necessitate dry needling or TrP injection: 1. persistent pain or discomfort after complete elimination of the underlying pathological lesion, 2. poor response to conservative therapy, 3. intolerable pain, 4. deep location of a TrP, rendering it inaccessible by conservative manual therapy, 5. inadequate time to accept the time-consuming conservative therapy, or 6. personal preference (25).

4. *Acute versus Chronic Myofascial Trigger Points*: In the acute stage, active TrPs are usually related to the defense mechanism to protect the acute traumatic lesion [pain to avoid overmovement that may interfere with the healing process], and should not be treated. However, in certain cases, inactivation of TrPs in the acute stage may be still necessary to control the intolerable pain.

5. *Superficial versus Deep Myofacial Trigger Points*: Deep pressure massage can be easily applied on the superficial TrPs, but not the deep ones. The deep TrPs may be treated much more easily with stretch, ultrasound, laser, acupressure, acupuncture, or local injection. Local TrP injection to a superficial TrP is much easier than the deep ones, since the taut band and focal tenderness [with pain recognition] can be palpated easily. Deep palpation of the TrP may facilitate needle penetration during TrP injection.

6. *Individual Preference [Patients and Clinicians]*: A patient who has needle-phobia may not accept TrP injection therapy. On the other hand, a patient who has a busy schedule may prefer to have TrP injection even though conservative physical therapy is effective to control the pain. A physician who is not familiar

with a special method [such as TrP injection] would prefer not to give such therapy.

7. *Other Considerations* include the availability of equipment or a device for a special treatment and the cost effective principle. If a patient with chronic pain feels better after physical therapy but the effectiveness lasts for only a short period and requires long-term therapy, the physician should try TrP injection since the effectiveness may last longer, and thus be less expensive than physical therapy.

Other Principles of Myofascial Pain Therapy include the elimination or treatment of perpetuation factors [if any], patient education, and appropriate home program.

PHYSICAL THERAPY FOR MYOFASCIAL PAIN

Manual Therapy: Manual therapy is an important category of myofascial pain therapy and has been described by various authorities (22-24,33,34). In general, the basic principles of manual therapy include stretching of shortening muscles [or taut band], improving local circulation, counter-irritation [stimulation to the nociceptors to cause reflex inhibition of pain-fiber conduction (35)], and certain mechanism via spinal reflexes [such as modification of TrP circuit (7)]. Frequently, the immediate effectiveness is obvious. However, the long-term effectiveness is still questionable.

Modalities: Although *thermotherapy* is not very effective to control myofascial pain, it is the most important modality to treat the soft tissue lesion since it can improve focal circulation to facilitate the healing process. It is suggested to apply heat before and after any treatment [including manual therapy, mechanical traction, electrotherapy, etc.]. Therapeutic ultrasound may also provide an additional mechanical energy directly to the TrPs. *Cold* application can provide temporary pain relief due to the effect of hyperstimulation analgesia. However, it usually induces vasoconstriction and impaired focal circulation. Therefore, cryotherapy is only recommended for TrP therapy during stretch of the tight muscles [stretching with intermittent cold application]. For temporary pain relief, *electrical nerve stimulation* [such as transcutaneous electrical nerve stimulation] is usually effective. For TrP therapy, *electrical muscle stimulation* is recommended, since the muscle contraction caused by the electrical stimulation is similar to focal massage (36). The mechanism of *laser therapy* on TrP is still unclear. It has been suggested that laser is a needleless [painless] acupuncture (37). Other methods for TrP therapy include iontophoresis, phonophoresis, traction device, vibration, movement therapy, biofeedback, etc. (22). A clinician can make a choice of any combination according to his own or the patient's preference. However, it should be based on a founded scientific wisdom.

MYOFASCIAL TRIGGER POINT INJECTION

General Principles of Myofascial Trigger Point Injection: Before considering TrP injection, the underlying etiological lesion should be treated and conservative treatment for the inactivation of the TrP should be tried. To determine which TrP would be injected, it is important to confirm that this TrP is the one to cause the discomfort [pain recognition] and to identify the key TrP. *During TrP injection*, the exact site of the TrP should be carefully located for needle penetration. A fingertip of the non-dominant hand should be placed over the TrP region to direct the location of the needle tip. The needle tip should encounter the sensitive loci in the TrP region to elicit LTR. It is essential to elicit LTR during TrP injection in order to obtain an immediate and complete relief of pain (1,25). A "fast-in and fast-out" technique is recommended for the needle penetration in order to avoid side movement of the needle with sharp edge and to provide high pressure to elicit LTRs (25). *After injection*, the sites of needle penetration in both skin and muscle should be compressed firmly for hemostasis. It has been found that excessive bleeding from the needle penetration may cause post-injection soreness (25). Cold packs can be applied over the injection sites only if there is evidence of severe active bleeding or hematoma formation. The injected muscle should be stretched to as full a range as possible after hemostasis. Thermotherapy can be applied on the site of injection after the stretch. Patient education including a home program should be re-emphasized after the procedure. The common causes of failure in TrP injection are listed in Table 2.

Fischer's Technique of Myofascial Trigger Point Injection: Fischer has recommended infiltrating the whole taut band including myotendonal junction during TrP injection (27,28). He has also developed a new technique, 'Pre-injection blocks,' to prevent pain which would be caused by needle penetration of sensitive tissue (27,28). The sensory nerves supplying the area to be injected are locally anesthetized prior to giving a TrP injection (27,28).

Injection of Botulinum Toxin: Botulinum toxin A can block acetylcholine release from the motor nerve ending and subsequently relieve the taut band in the TrP region. Several authors have demonstrated the efficacy of TrP injection with botulinum toxin A to control TrP pain (38,39). In an animal study, end plate noise recorded in the TrP region were suppressed after the injection of botulinum toxin A (40).

ACUPUNCTURE AND OTHER DRY NEEDLING THERAPIES

It has been demonstrated that acupuncture or dry needling of TrPs is effective for pain relief (41-49). However, it may increase the incidence of post-needling soreness (25). The simi- larity between dry needling and acupuncture has been documented (6,41-45). Melzack has suggested that 71 percent of TrPs are actually acupuncture points (35). The referred pain patterns of some TrPs are similar to the acupuncture meridian (6,7). Many authors have indicated the importance to elicit LTRs [similar to "De-Qui" or "The-Chi" effect in acupuncture] during needling in order to obtain an immediate and complete pain relief (1,6,7,25,42-45). It is possible that the strong pressure stimulation to the TrP units can provide very strong neural impulses to the dorsal horn cells in the spinal cord to break the vicious cycle of the TrP circuit (7).

Intramuscular stimulation has been used for myofascial pain therapy by Gunn since 1976 (47). Gunn uses an acupuncture needle for intramuscular stimulation therapy (45,46). Since the acupuncture needle is too flexible and hard to handle, Chu (42) uses an electromyography needle to perform dry needling with an attempt to obtain LTRs, so that she renames this procedure as "twitch-obtaining intramuscular stimulation." Both Gunn and Chu apply multiple needle insertions into the TrP region. Recently Chu further modified the technique by adding electrical stimulation during therapy, and giving a new name, "electrical twitch-obtaining intramuscular stimulation" (43,44).

Baldry applies the needle into the subcutaneous, but not the muscle tissue [superficial dry needling] (41). Goddard et al. (50) has demonstrated that superficial dry needling [sham acupuncture] has similar effect on pain relief as intramuscular needling [traditional acupuncture].

In recent reviews by Cummings and White (51), it was found that needling of TrPs appears to be an effective treatment. However, no trials in the 23 papers reviewed were of sufficient quality or design to test the efficacy of needling beyond placebo for myofascial pain. Controlled trials are required to further investigate this issue.

TABLE 2. Causes of Failure in Myofascial Trigger Point Injection

A. Technical Factors
1. No **precise location** of loci in a TrP region–no **LTR** elicited during injection.
2. Incomplete inactivation of **all sensitive loci** in a TrP region.
3. Excessive **damage** to muscle fibers, nerve fibers, or vessels.
4. Inadequate **hemostasis** after injection.

B. Diagnostic Factors
1. Inappropriate diagnosis and/or treatment of the **etiological lesions**.
2. Inappropriate determination of a primary TrP [**pain recognition**]
3. **Unreliable information** from patients [pain location, intensity, etc.].
4. Inappropriate evaluation and control of **perpetuating factors**.
5. **Long-standing** or **chronic** myofascial pain syndrome.
6. Superimposed **fibromyalgia** syndrome.
7. **Neurogenic pain, central pain or psychogenic pain.**

C. Aftercare Factors
1. Inappropriate [excessive, inadequate, or inaccurate] **medical care** including medication, physical therapy, alternative medicine, etc.
2. Inappropriate **home program**.
3. Inappropriate **physical and/or mental activity** including posture, daily living activity, working status [body mechanics, working environment, etc.], exercise, recreation, social activity, etc.

TrP = myofascial trigger point
LTR = local twitch response

REFERENCES

1. Hong C-Z: Lidocaine injection versus dry needling to myofascial trigger point: The importance of the local twitch response. Amer J Phys Med Rehabil 73: 256-263, 1994.

2. Hong C-Z: Persistence of local twitch response with loss of conduction to and from the spinal cord. Arch Phys Med Rehabil 75:12-16, 1994.

3. Hong C-Z: Pathophysiology of myofascial trigger point. J Formos Med Assoc 95:93-104, 1996.

4. Hong C-Z: Algometry in evaluation of trigger points and referred pain. J Musculoske Pain 6(1):47-59, 1998.

5. Hong C-Z: Current research on myofascial trigger points: Pathophysiological studies. J Musculoske Pain 7(1/2):121-129, 1999.

6. Hong C-Z: Myofascial trigger points: Pathophysiology and correlation with acupuncture points. Acup Med 18:41-47, 2000.

7. Hong C-Z: New Trends in Myofascial Pain Syndrome (Invited review). Chinese Medical Journal (Taipei) 65:501-512, 2002.

8. Hong C-Z, Chen J-T, Chen S-M, Yan J-J, Su Y-J: Histological findings of responsive loci in a myofascial trigger spot of rabbit skeletal muscle from where localized twitch responses could be elicited. Arch Phys Med Rehabil 77:962, 1996.

9. Hong C-Z, Simons DG: Pathophysiologic and electrophysiologic mechanism of myofascial trigger points. Arch Phys Med Rehabil 79:863-872, 1998.

10. Hong C-Z, Torigoe Y: Electrophysiologic characteristics of localized twitch responses in responsive bands of rabbit skeletal muscle fibers. J Musculoske Pain 2(2):17-43, 1994.

11. Hong C-Z, Torigoe Y, Yu J: The localized twitch responses in responsive bands of rabbit skeletal muscle fibers are related to the reflexes at spinal cord level. J Musculoske Pain 3(1):15-33, 1995.

12. Hubbard DR: Chronic and recurrent muscle pain: pathophysiology and treatment, and review of pharmacologic studies. J Musculoske Pain 4(1/2):123-143, 1996.

13. Mense S: Nociception from skeletal muscle in relation to clinical muscle pain. Pain 54:241-289, 1993.

14. Mense S: Peripheral mechanisms of muscle nociception and local muscle pain. J Musculoske Pain 1(1):133-170, 1993.

15. Mense S: Biochemical pathogenesis of myofascial pain. J Musculoske Pain 4(1/2):145-162, 1996.

16. Pongratz D: Neure Ergebnisse zur Pathogeneses Myofaszialer Schmerzsyndrome. Nervenheilkunde 21(1):35-37, 2002

17. Simons DG: Clinical and etiological update of myofascial pain from trigger points. J Musculoske Pain 4(1/2):93-121, 1996.

18. Simons DG: Diagnostic criteria of myofascial pain caused by trigger points. J Musculoske Pain 7(1/2):111-120, 1999.

19. Simons DG: Do endplate noise and spikes arise from normal motor endplates? Am J Phys Med Rehabil 80:134-140, 2001.

20. Simons DG, Hong C-Z, Simons LS: Prevalence of spontaneous electrical activity at trigger spots and at control sites in rabbit skeletal muscle. J Musculoske Pain 3(1):35-48, 1995.

21. Simons DG, Hong C-Z, Simons LS: Endplate potentials are common to midfiber myofascial trigger points. Am J Phys Med Rehabil 81:212-222, 2002.

22. Simons DG, Travell JG, Simons LS: Travell & Simons's myofascial pain and dysfunction: the trigger point manual. Vol. 1, 2nd ed., Baltimore: Williams & Wilkins, 1999.

23. Travell JG, Simons DG: Myofascial pain and dysfunction: The trigger point manual. Vol. 1. Baltimore: Williams & Wilkins, 1983.

24. Travell JG, Simons DG: Myofascial pain and dysfunction: The trigger point manual. Vol. 2. Baltimore: Williams & Wilkins, 1992.

25. Hong C-Z: Consideration and recommendation of myofascial trigger point injection. J Musculoske Pain 2(1):29-59, 1994.

26. Borg-Stein J, Simons DG: Myofascial pain. Arch Phys Med Rehabil 83: (Suppl 1):S40-47, 2002.

27. Fischer AA: New approach in treatment of myofascial pain. Phys Med Rehab Clinic North America 8(1):153-169, 1997.

28. Fischer AA: Treatment of myofascial pain. J Musculoske Pain 7(1/2):131-142, 1999.

29. Hong C-Z, Jou EM, Kuan T-S, Chen S-M, Chen J-T: The management of Myofascial Trigger Points. J Rehab Med Assoc ROC 31:67-77, 2003.

30. Hsueh T-C, Yu S, Kuan T-S, Hong C-Z: Association of active myofascial trigger points and cervical disc lesion. J Formos Med Assoc 97:174-180, 1998.

31. Bogduk N, Simons DG: Neck pain: Joint pain or trigger points? In: Progress in Fibromyalgia and Myofascial Pain, Chapter 20, pp. 267-73, Vol 6 of Pain research and clinical management. Ed. Vaeroy H, Mersky H. Elsevier, Amsterdam, 1993.

32. Lee P-S, Lin P, Hsieh L-F, Hong C-Z: Facet injection to control the recurrent myofascial trigger points: A case report. J Rehab Med Assoc ROC 26:41-45, 1998.

33. Kostopoulos D, Rizopoulos K: The manual of trigger point and myofascial therapy. SLACK Incorporated, Thorofare, New Jersey, 2001.

34. Kraft GH [consulting editor], Stanton DF, Mein EA [Guest Editors]: Manual Medicine. Physical Medicine and Rehabilitation Clinic of North America, 7(4): 679-932, 1996.

35. Melzack R: Myofascial trigger points: Relation to acupuncture and mechanism of pain. Arch Phys Med Rehabil 62:114-117, 1981.

36. Hsueh T-C, Cheng P-T, Kuan T-S, Hong C-Z: The immediate effectiveness of electrical nerve stimulation on myofascial trigger points. Am J Phys Med Rehabil 76:471-476, 1997.

37. Kleinkort JA, Foley RA: Laser Acupuncture: Its Use in Physical Therapy. Am J Acupuncture 12:51-56, 1984.

38. Cheshire WP, Abashian SW, Mann JD: Botulinum toxin in the treatment of myofascial pain syndrome. Pain 59:65-69,1994.

39. Wheeler AH, Goolkasian P, Gretz SS: A randomized, double-blind, prospective pilot study of Botulinum

toxin injection for refractory, unilateral, cervicothoracic, paraspinal, myofascial pain syndrome. Spine 23: 1662-1667, 1998.

40. Kuan T-S, Chen J-T, Chen S-M, Chen C-H, Hong C-Z: Effect of Botulinum toxin on endplate noise in myofascial trigger spots of rabbit skeletal muscle. Am J Phys Med Rehabil 81:512-520, 2002.

41. Baldry PE: Superficial dry needling. In: Fibromyalgia syndrome: A practitioner's guide to treatment. CL Chaitow (Ed.). Churchill Livingston, Edinburgh. 2000.

42. Chu J: Twitch-obtaining intramuscular stimulation: observation in the management of radiculopathic chronic low back pain. J Musculoske Pain 7(4):131-146, 1999.

43. Chu J, Neuhauser D, Schwartz I, et al.: The efficacy of automated/electrical twitch-obtaining intramuscular stimulation (ATOIMS/ETOIMS) for chronic pain control: Evaluation with statistical process control methods. Electromyogr Clin Neurophysiol 42:393-401, 2002.

44. Chu J, Yuen K, Wang B, Chang RC, Schwartz I, Neuhauser D: Elelctrical twitch-obtaining intramuscular stimulation in lower back pain. Am J Phys Med Rehabil 83:104-111, 2004.

45. Gunn CC: Treatment of chronic pain. Intramuscular stimulation for myofascial pain of radiculopathic origin. Churchill Livingston, London, UK, 1996.

46. Gunn CC: Radiculopathic pain: Diagnosis and treatment of segmental irritation or sensitization. J Musculoske Pain 5(4):119-134, 1997.

47. Gunn CC, Milbrandt WE: Tenderness at motor points—A diagnostic and prognostic aid for low back injury. J Bone Joint Surg 58:815-825, 1976.

48. Irnich D, Behrens N, Gleditsch JM, Stor W, Schreiber MA, Schops P, Vicker AJ, Beyer A: Immediate effects of dry needling and acupuncture at distant points in the chronic neck pain: Results of a randomized, double-blind, sham-controlled crossover trial. Pain 99: 83-89, 2002

49. Lewit K: The needle effect in relief of myofascial pain. Pain 6:83-90, 1979.

50. Goddard G, Karibe H, McNeill C, Vallafuerte E: Acupuncture and sham acupuncture reduce muscle pain in the myofascial pain patients. Orofac Pain 16(1):71-76, 2002.

51. Cummings TM, White AR: Needling therapies in the management of myofascial trigger point pain: A systemic review. Arch Phys Med Rehabil 82:986-992, 2001.

Pain and the Neuroendocrine System

Gunther Neeck

Acute pain of a distinct intensity acts as an acute stressor and induces neuroendocrine reactions. It has become increasingly evident that the hypothalamus-hypophysis-adrenal cortex axis [HPA] plays a central role in the stress response to painful and other stimuli. Activation of neurons which produce the corticotrophin-releasing hormone [CRH] in the hypothalamus stimulates the axis hypophysis-adrenal cortex. Chronic pain leads via CRH and via, e.g., the hypothalamic somatostatin, to a whole concert of hypothalamic-hypophyseal interactions with a permanent effect on the regulation of peripheral glands, too. These alterations are accompanied by numerous dysfunctions of the autonomous nervous system. Acute stress of high intensity, e.g., after severe trauma, induces analgesia via activation of the pain-inhibiting [antinociceptive] system. Chronic stress reduces the pain threshold on the level of the central nervous system by an activation of the pain-facilitating [pronociceptive] pathways. So the interactions between pain and the neuroendocrine system are bidirectional.

Gunther Neeck, MD, PhD, is affiliated with the Department of Internal Medicine and Center of Rheumatology, Rostock Clinic South, Suedring 81, 18059 Rostock, Germany.

[Haworth co-indexing entry note]: "Pain and the Neuroendocrine System." Neeck, Gunther. Co-published simultaneously in *Journal of Musculoskeletal Pain* [The Haworth Medical Press, an imprint of The Haworth Press, Inc.] Vol. 12, No. 3/4, 2004, p. 45; and: *Soft Tissue Pain Syndromes: Clinical Diagnosis and Pathogenesis* [ed: Dieter E. Pongratz, Siegfried Mense, and Michael Spaeth] The Haworth Medical Press, an imprint of The Haworth Press, Inc., 2004, p. 45. Single or multiple copies of this article are available for a fee from The Haworth Document Delivery Service [1-800-HAWORTH, 9:00 a.m. - 5:00 p.m. [EST]. E-mail address: docdelivery@haworthpress.com].

doi:10.1300/J094v12n03_07

Developments in the Fibromyalgia Syndrome

I. Jon Russell

SUMMARY. Objectives: The goals of this presentation are to document contemporary views and new information about the fibromyalgia syndrome [FMS].

Findings: As the FMS becomes better known and understood, it is increasingly important that agreement be achieved on classification and terminology relating to it and other conditions with which it might be confused. The term "soft tissue pain" is recommended as a general heading for a variety of pain syndromes that involve muscles, nerves, ligaments, tendons and bursae. The American College of Rheumatology research classification for FMS has been critical to the rapid progress in understanding this disorder but there is understandable agitation to develop a clinical case definition [CCD] that can be appropriately applied to community medical practice. It is easier to suggest a CCD than to accomplish the necessary validation study. Many objective physiological and biochemical abnormalities have been described in FMS patients and some have been confirmed by several independent investigators. It is not yet clear which of these should be considered etiologic in its development versus the result of living with chronic pain and insomnia. Genetic subgroups would certainly seem to indicate a genetic predisposition to develop FMS. The management of FMS seems to be improving considerably. Medications are now being shown to correct objective abnormalities. Medications developed to manage neuropathic pain are being prospectively tested in FMS with hopes of achieving formal indication for this condition.

Conclusions: The FMS is no longer unknown to the medical practitioner. This new status requires practical diagnostic criteria validated for use in community care, a common nomenclature, a better understanding of pathogenesis, and effective treatment modalities. Remarkably, there is dramatic progress in all of these areas. *[Article copies available for a fee from The Haworth Document Delivery Service: 1-800-HAWORTH. E-mail address: <docdelivery@haworthpress.com> Website: <http://www.HaworthPress.com> © 2004 by The Haworth Press, Inc. All rights reserved.]*

KEYWORDS. Fibromyalgia syndrome, classification, soft tissue pain, pathogenesis, treatment

Over the past three years, there has been substantial progress in the recognition and understanding of the fibromyalgia syndrome [FMS]. This progress is acknowledged to have been in the categories of diagnosis, pathogenesis, and management. The present review will attempt to highlight a few of the issues regarding the current status in these three areas. It is acknowledged that the approach taken to the issues in each category is not uniform nor comprehen-

I. Jon Russell, MD, PhD, is Associate Professor of Medicine, Division of Clinical Immunology, and Director, University Clinical Research Center, University of Texas Health Science Center, San Antonio, TX, USA; Editor, *Journal of Musculoskeletal Pain*; International Pain Consultant to Pain Research & Management, *The Journal of the Canadian Pain Society*, London, ON, Canada; Editorial Board Member of *Pain Watch*; and Honorary Board Member, Lupus Foundation of America.

[Haworth co-indexing entry note]: "Developments in the Fibromyalgia Syndrome." Russell. I. Jon. Co-published simultaneously in *Journal of Musculoskeletal Pain* [The Haworth Medical Press, an imprint of The Haworth Press, Inc.] Vol. 12. No. 3/4. 2004, pp. 47-57; and: *Soft Tissue Pain Syndromes: Clinical Diagnosis and Pathogenesis* [ed: Dieter E. Pongratz. Siegfried Mense. and Michael Spaeth] The Haworth Medical Press. an imprint of The Haworth Press, Inc.. 2004. pp. 47-57. Single or multiple copies of this article are available for a fee from The Haworth Document Delivery Service [1-800-HAWORTH, 9:00 a.m. - 5:00 p.m. [EST]. E-mail address: docdelivery@haworthpress.com].

Available online at http://www.haworthpress.com/web/JMP
© 2004 by The Haworth Press, Inc. All rights reserved.
doi:10.1300/J094v12n03_08

sive. In addition, the content addressed under each topic reflects the author's philosophy about definable progress. The limited space available necessitates a more cryptic approach than would be ideal.

DIAGNOSIS

It is important to the diagnosis and characterization of the fibromyalgia syndrome [FMS] that physicians in practice, physicians in training, even patients with FMS, know where FMS fits in the spectrum of disorders that can cause body pain.

Errant Terminology

Some physicians improperly refer to a wide range of conditions generically as "myofascial pain" and imply that they all exhibit "trigger points". Others have continued to use the term non-articular rheumatism. Use of the term "myofascial pain" generically is problematic because there is a specific regional pain condition called the "myofascial pain syndrome" [MPS]. It is characterized by spontaneous soft tissue pain at trigger points [TrPs] in skeletal muscles, irritability of muscle fibers to stimulate that produce a taut band, referral of discomfort to a reproducible zone of reference, and limited range of motion (1,2). Misuse of the term trigger points often occurs in reference to places where the patient is tender to deep palpation pressure, inappropriately lumping together tendinitis, bursitis, true TrPs and the tender points [TePs] of FMS. Non-articular rheumatism is an antiquated term traditionally applied by rheumatologists to inflammatory pain and tenderness in soft tissue in conditions like tendinitis and bursitis.

Soft Tissue Pain Classification

It is now recommended that the term "Soft Tissue Pain [STP] syndromes" be adopted as the generic name for a logical classification of these disorders [see Table 1]. The classification includes only three subcategories to encompass localized, regionalized, and generalized STP disorders. A simple body pain diagram, completed by the patient in the waiting room, may

TABLE 1. Classification of Soft Tissue Pain Disorders

Classification of Soft Tissue Pain [STP] Disorders (1,2)

Localized:
a. Bursitis [subacromial, olecranon, trochanteric, prepatellar, anserine]
b. Tenosynovitis [biceps, supraspinatus, infrapatellar, Achilles]
c. Enthesopathy [39 total, lateral epicondylitis, medial epicondylitis]
d. Entrapment Syndrome [carpal tunnel, tarsal tunnel, cubital tunnel]

Regionalized:
a. Myofascial Pain Syndrome [MPS, e.g., piriformis, iliopsoas, trapezius]
b. Masticatory Myofascial Pain Syndrome [TMJ, TMD]
c. Referred Pain [angina or subphrenic abscess to shoulder, hip to thigh]
d. Complex Regional Pain Syndrome [CRPS]
   i Type 1–non-trauma [replaces reflex sympathetic dystrophy]
   ii Type 2–trauma [replaces causalgia]

Generalized:
a. Polymyalgia Rheumatica   [PMR] [can also be arthritic]
b. Hypermobility Syndrome   [HMS]
c. Fibromyalgia Syndrome   [FMS]
d. Chronic Fatigue Syndrome [CFS] when painful [WSP]

be all that is needed to guide the physician to the proper diagnostic subcategory [see Figure 1]. The simple abbreviation "STP" can easily be used in the doctor's notes to indicate a category of information from the medical history and the relevant findings on physical examination.

Most of the "localized" conditions, such as bursitis and tendinitis and some of the enthesopathies, are believed to result from repetitive mechanical injury to inadequately conditioned tissues. They are often named anatomically and are disclosed by a typical history plus the exquisite tenderness elicited by digital palpation of the affected structures.

The "regionalized" syndromes can also result from "overuse," and may involve more than one type of body structure. Despite that, they are limited in anatomic scope to a region or body quadrant. The MPS described above encompasses a family of regionalized conditions characterized by TrPs in skeletal muscles, which behave differently than the TePs, of FMS. The masticatory myofascial pain dysfunction syndromes [MPDS] comprise another family of conditions of the head and neck that can involve a dysfunctional temporomandibular joint and/ or TrPs in the muscles of mastication. Several types of visceral pain can be referred to a single musculoskeletal structure or to a region of the body [eg., angina felt in the shoulder or jaw].

FIGURE 1. Four body pain diagrams [a. left subacromial bursitis; b. left myofascial pain syndrome; c. and d. fibromyalgia syndrome].

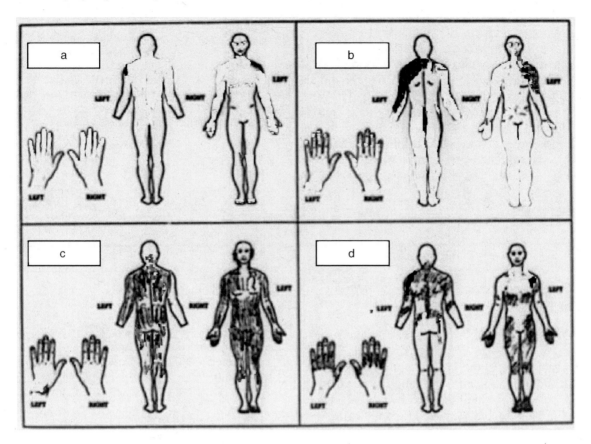

The recently renamed complex regional pain syndromes [CRPS Type 1 and Type 2, formerly, reflex sympathetic dystrophy and causalgia, respectively] would be classified in this category as well.

In the "Generalized" category the term "widespread pain" [WSP] is best illustrated by FMS patients who report of "pain all over." This category also includes the chronic fatigue syndrome [CFS] when that condition is painful.

The main purpose of discussing classification in this setting is to emphasize that it is easier to communicate when we all use the same language. On the other hand, the classification also speaks to pathogenesis, since the mechanisms responsible for generalized pain are more likely to involve a systemic process than are conditions that present as localized or regionalized conditions.

Research Classification of the Fibromyalgia Syndrome

In 1990, the American College of Rheumatology [ACR] (3) approved the ACR criteria for research classification of the FMS. The purpose at the time was to acknowledge the existence of a syndrome and to help investigators to judge the admissibility of a given individual with body pain as a candidate for FMS research. There have been concerns about the growing use of these research criteria for clinical diagnosis in settings for which they were not validated (4).

Canadian Clinical Case Definition of the Fibromyalgia Syndrome

A Canadian fibromyalgia action group achieved the approval of Health Canada to explore new criteria for the diagnosis of FMS in the clinical community. What they came up with is the ACR Criteria based on pain/tenderness but modified by a number of other systemic manifestations characteristic of FMS (5). The resultant Clinical Case Definition of FMS is intended to prompt the clinician to recognize a wider syndrome pattern than the one limited to pain/tenderness and to take non-pain factors into consideration in the treatment of FMS. Of course, it is acknowledged that these criteria must be validated in the community clinical setting before they can be officially used with the idea that their operating characteristics are known.

PATHOGENESIS

Subgroups versus Overlap Fibromyalgia Syndromes

It has become increasingly relevant to discussions of FMS pathogenesis to consider the possibility that the FMS is not homogeneous. Rather, FMS seems to be composed of a number of related conditions which are all identified clinically by the same research classification criteria (3). It is as if a few distinct initiating factors, working in fertile environments, have initiated processes that eventually follow the same [or a similar] final common pathway to produce the clinical features now recognized as FMS. The illustration in Figure 2 shows a hypothetical model of a sequence of events which begins with one or more predisposing factors acted upon, at some point in time, by an event or agent, to initiate a sequence of events which involve chemical changes in the central nervous system. The neurochemical abnormalities understandably lead to clinical manifestations that result in a compromised individual with chronic clinical and emotional findings.

Differences in the initiating pathogenesis of FMS subgroups could be responsible for the observed heterogeneity with respect to clinical presentation, to neurochemical abnormalities, and to responsiveness to potent medications. For example, one research group (6,7) distinguishes people meeting ACR criteria for the research classification of FMS (3) into two clinical groups: those who have sought care for their

FIGURE 2. A hypothetical model showing a sequence of events leading to the fibromyalgia syndrome. The sequence begins with one or more predisposing factors acted upon at some point in time by an event or agent to initiate a sequence of events which involve neurochemical changes in the central nervous system. The neurochemical abnormalities understandably lead to clinical manifestations that cause collateral damage in many clinical systems. The result is a very compromised individual with chronic clinical and emotional findings.

Proposed Pathogenesis Model

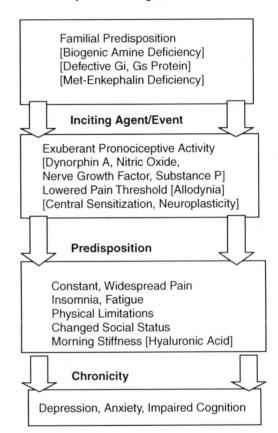

pain are called "FMS patients" while those who have not sought care are called "FMS non-patients". The point is that they then find a number of clinical and biological differences between these subpopulations.

Similarly, about half of the FMS patients in a study of antipolymer antibodies exhibited elevated levels while the others did not (8). In a treatment study (9), about 50 percent of the FMS patients responded beneficially to ketamine while the others did not. The FMS that is comorbid with rheumatoid arthritis [RA] in about one third of RA patients was considered to be clinically indistinguishable from primary FMS but the two conditions can be distinguished by the presence of elevated nerve growth factor [NGF] in the cerebrospinal fluid [CSF] of only the primary FMS patients (10).

The viewpoint of the observer can have an important influence in how FMS patients are perceived. Clinicians would generally prefer to be lumpers, hoping that the limited therapeutic resources available to them will work similarly in all of the apparently similar conditions. By contrast, students of pathogenesis would rather be splitters, hoping to have the subgroup under study be as homogeneous as possible before seeking evidence for specific patterns of pathophysiology and/or pathochemistry that most of the affected individuals have in common.

Pure as Possible for Pathogenesis [3Ps]

If the pathogenesis is different for different subgroups of FMS, it seems only logical that we should try to try to distinguish subgroups of FMS for the purpose of research study and include, for each study group, the most homogeneous combination of participants possible. I think of this as a plea for adherence to the three "Ps" of bio-clinical research; "Pure as Possible for Pathogenesis." If one is successful in picking a very homogeneous study group, there should be an amplification of the biochemical abnormalities [less dilution of biochemical markers by the presence of dissimilar individuals] and stronger correlations with the relevant clinical manifestation of that biochemical phenotype. One way of accomplishing this homogeneity in retrospect is to examine post-hoc the subgroup of individuals identified by the presence of a measured marker and then to characterize that subgroup on the basis of clinical phenotype. That knowledge of a subgroup's clinical phenotype will facilitate future attempts to prospectively seek the clinical phenotype as a marker of subgroup and could be expected to confirm the biological abnormality as validation of the clinical selection process.

This could appear to represent circular reasoning, but, in fact, it is a methodology by which quantum leaps can be made in the face of a confusing syndrome composed of different subgroups that exhibit the same final common pathway. This concept can be illustrated by the historical value of the Fredrickson classification of lipoprotein disorders (11), in which the final common manifestation was death by myocardial infarction. It was learned, however, that specific treatment of subgroups for the unique defect identified would improve the overall mortality of lipid disorders one subgroup at a time. That kind of focused benefit would have been much more difficult to achieve without the benefit of a biochemical classification.

Depression–Biological Markers, Antipolymer Antibodies, and Cytokines

In the past, there have been intermittent reports of lymphocyte immune abnormalities in people with FMS but the outcomes of the studies were quite variable and hard to interpret in light of the clinical picture (12). More recently, two studies have critically evaluated the possible role of cytokines in patients with FMS (13,14). While most of the cytokines explored in these investigations did not differ between FMS and HNC, there were some dramatic, consistent, and relevant exceptions. The serum interleukin-8 [IL-8] and the interleukin-6 [IL-6] from in vitro stimulated PBMC cultures were significantly higher for the FMS subjects. There were also correlates with comorbidities. The serum IL-8 was most dramatically elevated in FMS patients who were also depressed, but it also correlated with pain intensity and the duration of FMS symptoms. Since IL-8 promotes sympathetic pain and IL-6 induces hyperalgesia, fatigue, and depression, it is hypothesized that they both may play a role in modulating the symptoms of FMS. Interleukin-8 is a monocyte derived 8.0 kiloDalton chemokine that promotes neutrophil chemotaxis and degranulation. Its signaling of other cells is mediated by high-affinity G protein-coupled receptors. Its production in vitro is stimulated by substance P, so that may help to explain the elevation of both of these cytokines even in different fluid compartments of FMS patients.

In this light, it is of interest that IL-6 has been successfully administered to people with FMS, with the finding that it substantially modulated the severity of the FMS-related symptoms (15). That experiment was undertaken because IL-6 can serve as a direct or at least indirect stimulus of the hypothalamic pituitary adrenal [HPA] axis but the effects on FMS patients were rather global. It is certainly possible that FMS is an IL-6 deficiency state and that the production of IL-6 by PBMC during in vitro culture bears no relationship to in vivo production of IL-6 where it is needed in the central nervous system.

Genetic Issues in Fibromyalgia Syndrome– 30 Percent Familial–Two Subgroups

Evidence for familial aggregation and a genetic basis for the disorder is receiving attention. About one third of FMS patients report that another family member, usually a female, has a similar, chronic pain condition, or has already been given the diagnosis of FMS (Russell, 1994, unpublished). Several published studies have documented familial patterns and some have predicted an autosomal dominant mode of inheritance for FMS (16,17). There is growing evidence for an autosomal dominant mode of inheritance for FMS (18). A recent genetic study (19) found probable linkage of FMS with the histocompatibility locus examined by the sibship method.

A complete genome scan of family members with two or more FMS affected members is currently underway (Olson J et al., 2004, unpublished) using samples of deoxyribonucleic acid [DNA] from a large number of FMS multicase families for comparison with clinical and laboratory genotypic features. Meanwhile, several candidate genes have been proposed to directly explain specific metabolic abnormalities that have been consistently observed in FMS.

In one such examination, 80 multicase FMS families were examined using a total of eight markers spanning the genomic regions for the serotonin transporter [HTTLPR, three regional markers] on chromosome 17; the serotonin receptor 2A [HTR2A, three regional markers] on chromosome 13; and the histocompatibility locus antigen [HLA, two regional markers] region of chromosome 6 (20). No evidence for linkage was found in the HTTLPR region. Families with an older age of onset were linked to the HLA region [lod = 3.02, P = .00057], suggesting an immune-mediated pathogenesis. In the HTR2A region, the results indicated a moderately strong linkage to families with a youn-

ger age of onset, less severe pain, lower levels of depression, and absence of the irritable bowel syndrome [lod = 5.56, P = .000057]. The HTR2A genome is polymorphically imprinted, so the issue of parent-of-origin will need to be considered in future studies. Bio-informatics mining and further sequencing of the genes in the HTR2A region will need to be utilized to identify specific polymorphisms for further clinical association testing.

Another appealing gene candidate for a role in causing FMS would be the catechol-O-methyltransferase [COMT] enzyme that physiologically inactivates catecholamines such as dopamine, norepinephrine, endorphins, and catecholamine-containing drugs. Polymorphism [really dimorphism] in the gene encodes for variations in the activity of the COMT enzyme. The COMT gene exists in two forms [L and H] which make copies differing by a single amino acid [either valine or methionine] at the variable site. This small variation has a big effect on the activity of COMT. Subjects with the LL phenotype, who have two copies of the methionine version, make three to four-fold less COMT than the HH variants, which contain valine at the variable site.

The significance of COMT polymorphism [LL, LH, or HH] in FMS was assessed by Gursoy and colleagues (21). The analysis of COMT polymorphism was performed using polymerase chain reaction [PCR]. Sixty-one patients with FMS and 61 HNC were included in the study. Although no significant difference was found between LL and LH separately, the LL and LH genotypes together were more highly represented in FMS patients than in the HNC [P = 0.024]. In addition, HH genotypes in FMS were significantly lower than in the HNC groups [P = 0.04]. There was no significant relationship between COMT polymorphism and the psychiatric status of the patients, as assessed by several psychiatric tests [P > 0.05].

It has been hypothesized (22) that COMT functions by metabolizing dopamine and freeing receptors in the brain for the binding of endorphins to the mu-opioid receptors, which lead to pain relief. The more potent the COMT enzyme that is functioning in the body the more dopamine that gets metabolized and more endorphins are allowed to bind. The LL genotype has been associated with increased pain susceptibility.

The findings of these and other studies of genetic linkage to FMS clinical patterns have provided strong support for the concept that there are subgroups of FMS which present with unique but overlapping clinical manifestations. It is likely that genetic characterization of FMS subgroups will do more than any of the previous clinical and laboratory studies to move FMS from its current classification as a "syndrome" to that of a "disease." If that is true, it will likely come at the expense of subdividing the currently large clinical population of FMS into many subgroups. The advantage may be that the pathogenesis of those subgroups will be more apparent and the development of strategic chemical therapies will be substantially facilitated.

G Protein Coupled Receptors [GPCRs]

A family of cell surface receptors, known as G protein coupled receptors, allow molecules on the outside of the cell membranes to signal their presence to the inside of the cell and to direct specific intracellular functions. When the effect is to be a stimulation, the receptor is designated a "Gs" protein coupled receptor. When the designated function is inhibition of an intracellular process, the receptor is known as a "Gi" protein coupled receptor. G protein coupled receptor systems are composed of several protein molecules interacting with each other at the level of the cell membrane [see Figure 3].

The G protein receptor itself is envisioned as having many folds with loops that cross the cell membrane many times, leaving folds of the protein both inside and outside of the cell. On the outside of the membrane, the external folds specifically interact with the ligand, while the folds on the inside of the membrane interact with the internal phosphorylation complex. The internal complex is composed of an alpha, a beta, a gamma and a delta subunit which then interact with the effector molecule. A cartoon available on line at the following address illustrates the process for a hormone specific receptor [http://www.tamu.edu/classes/bich/eharris/411/Tutorials/1].

In the case of both the Gi and Gs protein coupled receptors, the effector molecule is the en-

FIGURE 3. G protein coupled receptor systems. This complex of several protein subunits can respond to an external ligand by stimulating [Gs, containing alpha s subunit] or inhibiting [Gi, containing alpha I subunit] the production of intracellular cyclic adenosine monophosphate by influencing the activity of the enzyme adenyl cyclase.

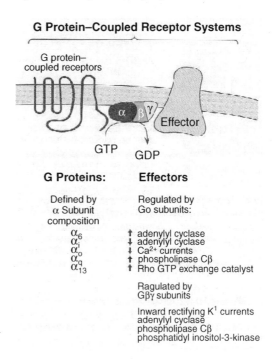

G Protein–Coupled Receptor Systems

G Proteins:
Defined by α Subunit composition

α_s
α_i
α_o
α_q
α_{13}

Effectors
Regulated by Go subunits:

↑ adenylyl cyclase
↓ adenylyl cyclase
↓ Ca²⁺ currents
↑ phospholipase Cβ
↑ Rho GTP exchange catalyst

Ragulated by Gβγ subunits

Inward rectifying K¹ currents
adenylyl cyclase
phospholipase Cβ
phosphatidyl inositol-3-kinase

zyme adenylcyclase which converts adenosine triphosphate [ATP] to cyclic adenosine monophosphate [cAMP]. The intracellular objective from Gs or Gi receptor activation is to regulate production of cAMP; Gs receptor activation increases intracellular cAMP by activating the intracellular enzyme adenylcyclase. By contrast, Gi receptor activation inhibits intracellular increases of cAMP by decreasing the activity of the intracellular enzyme adenylcyclase. One of the characteristics of certain Gi protein coupled receptors is their ability to be blocked or inactivated by pertussis toxoid. Similarly, the functions of many Gs protein coupled receptors can be blocked by cholera toxin.

Investigators in Florence, Italy performed a controlled experiment involving peripheral blood mononuclear cells [PBMC] from healthy normal controls [HNC] and from FMS patients (23). They used forskolin to non-specifically stimulate cAMP production by the cells and used the non-hydrolysable analogue of guanosine triphosphate [GTP] guanilyl-5′-imidophosphate [Gpp[NH]p] in a range of doses to progressively activate the inhibitory effect of the Gi protein coupled receptor.

They preincubated some of the HNC cells with pertussis toxoid to inactivate [poison] the Gi protein-coupled receptor in those cells. When forskolin and Gpp[NH]p were added to untreated HNC cells, production of cAMP was inhibited. When forskolin and Gpp[NH]p were added to pertussis toxoid treated HNC cells, the normal inhibition of cAMP production did not occur. When untreated [without pertussis toxoid exposure] FMS cells were stimulated with forskolin in the presence of Gpp[NH]p, they failed to inhibit cAMP in the same way as occurred with the poisoned HNC. This defect has been proposed to be a sufficient cause for the allodynia that is so characteristic of FMS.

Another group of investigators (24), working in the dental school at the University of California at Los Angeles, examined the function of a Gs protein coupled receptor in the PBMC of FMS patients and documented a defect in the response of that receptor to a beta-adrenergic ligand. To investigate the function of that receptor, PBMC from female FMS patients were compared with the functions of nine demographically-matched HNC. Aliquots of cells were incubated with or without stimulation by the beta-agonist isoproterenol. Basal and stimulated intracellular cAMP levels were determined by enzyme immunoassay. Two different concentrations of the isoproterenol [10^{-3} M and 10^{-5} M] were utilized. The basal levels of cAMP in FMS patients were numerically but not significantly elevated compared with the HNC. By contrast, isoproterenol, at 10^{-5} M, significantly increased cAMP in the HNC cells, but did not increase the mean intracellular cAMP levels in the FMS PBMC. The authors concluded that these preliminary results imply diminished Gs protein coupled beta adrenergic receptor function in FMS.

These two "first of their kind experiments in FMS" were performed to seek dysfunction in different G protein coupled receptors that target cAMP second messenger production in FMS PBMC. The fact that both experiments were successful is of some concern because it is difficult to explain involvement of two receptors from different genetic locations and with opposite effects on the same second messenger. Both types of experiments need to be independently confirmed. Is it possible that both types of receptors suffer from a common defect in FMS? The G protein coupled receptors are composed of several protein subunits. The Gi or Gs designations are based on the alpha component of each receptor. Perhaps there is a defect in one of the other components that is common to both groups of receptors. Alternatively, it is also possible that the alpha component of both the Gi and Gs suffers from a similar defect which is being measured as two defects because of the experimental designs.

MANAGEMENT

Medications

It is expected that the development of new drugs will bring more effective treatment that can be strategically applied earlier in the course of FMS. Several such medications, with possible roles in the management of FMS, were not close to availability three years ago but are now available.

Tizanidine–Alpha-2-Adrenergic Agonist

Tizanidine [Zanaflex®] is a central alpha-2 adrenergic agonist which should have an effect on the descending inhibition pathway of the spinal cord and has the potential to reduce the elevated levels of cerebrospinal fluid [CSF] substance P [SP]. An open-label, dose-titration study was conducted with a laboratory measure [CSF SP by radioimmunoassay] as the primary outcome variable. Spinal fluid was obtained before therapy and again on therapy after taking the medication for two months. The average CSF SP level fell significantly during therapy and several secondary measures showed clinical benefits. It was concluded that tizanidine treatment of FMS patients produced a significant reduction in CSF SP and clinical improvement. It should be noted that transaminitis developed in 20 percent so continuous therapy with this drug should be carefully monitored with laboratory tests.

Duloxetine–A Serotonin Norepinephrine Reuptake Inhibitor [SNRI]

Duloxetine was studied in FMS patients with and without depression. Significant improvement in several clinical measures were reported. Improvements were seen regardless of depression status at baseline. Side effects were generally benign.

Milnacipran–A Norepinephrine Serotonin Reuptake Inhibitor [NSRI]

Milnacipran-treated patients also improved in several of the typical FMS clinical symptoms with a paucity of adverse effects to limit its use.

Pregabalin–Alpha-2-Delta Receptor Agonist

This anticonvulsant drug has been reported to raise the firing threshold of central neurons, which may be the mechanism of benefit in patients with FMS. There have been several clinical trials of this agent to assess its efficacy and safety for reducing pain and associated symptoms in patients with FMS. Pregabalin-treated patients experienced significant improvement in subjective pain and improved sleep. The most common adverse experiences were dizziness and drowsiness.

Human Growth Hormone [HGH]

Growth hormone was studied because it was known to be produced during delta wave sleep, which many FMS patients fail to achieve normally. Growth hormone is difficult to measure because its release is pulsatile and its plasma half life is very short. An alternative means of monitoring growth hormone production has been to measure the plasma levels of insulin-like growth factor-1 [IGF1] which has a long half life. An age-adjusted deficiency of IGF1 has been documented in a large number of FMS patients relative to normal controls (25).

In one well-designed study, parenteral therapy [daily injections] with HGH was effective in reducing the severity of FMS symptoms (26) but regular injection therapy with this hormone is not universally appealing to FMS patients, IGF1 levels must be regularly monitored to adjust the HGH dosage, and the cost of such therapy is currently prohibitive. Deficient function of the growth hormone axis could contribute to symptoms in FMS patients, particularly decreased psychological well-being and reduced exercise capacity.

Pyridostigmine–For Growth Hormone Secretion During Exercise

Another insight is that HGH is normally produced during exercise but FMS patients fail to produce HGH during aerobic exercise (27). It was proposed that the release of HGH during exercise might be suppressed in FMS by somatostatin and that administration of pyridostigmine before exercise can disinhibit HGH production. Indeed, 30 mg of pyridostigmine, given before exercise resulted in increased release of HGH with exercise among FMS patients. It will be interesting to await the long-term studies of FMS exercise facilitated by pre-exercise dosing FMS patients with 30 mg of pyridostigmine or by daily therapy using 60 mg of sustained release pyridostigmine. Certainly, both of those approaches will be less expensive than parenteral replacement of HGH.

Surgery May Be Excessive in Fibromyalgia Syndrome

A study from South Africa (28) assessed the impact of spinal surgery in patients with FMS and back pain. The study patients with known FMS present with neck and/or back pain. They were evaluated with diagnostic techniques [e.g., magnetic resonance imaging] and had spinal surgery to correct "abnormalities" [e.g., "disc prolapse"]. The study used a retrospective design over a two year period to assess the outcome of surgery. Of the 50 respondents, 60 percent had neck surgery, 50 percent had lower back surgery, and 62 percent had more than one spinal operation. Over half of respondents experienced little or no improvement in pain scores or were worse in the six-12 months after spinal surgery. A similar proportion reported that they would not again select surgery as a modality of treatment. The authors concluded that FMS patients with back/neck pain must be evaluated with circumspection before spinal surgery is recommended. When surgery is performed, optimal analgesia during and after the procedure may be imperative to prevent central sensitization.

NATURAL HISTORY OF FIBROMYALGIA SYNDROME– CAUSES OF DEATH

There has been very little study of the causes of death in people with FMS. A recently completed study addressed this issue in Danish patients with FMS (29). Patients who were referred to a university hospital with a presumptive diagnosis of FMS [N = 1,361] were followed during the period of 1984-1999. The cohort was followed for a total of 5,295 person-years at risk and linked to the Danish Mortality Register. The investigators detected an increased risk of death from suicide, liver cirrhosis/biliary tract disease, and cerebrovascular disease. The causes of the increased rate of suicide in FMS were not disclosed but increased rates of lifetime depression, anxiety, and psychiatric disorders were likely contributors. The authors proposed that the risk factors for suicide should be sought at time of diagnosis and with each subsequent follow up visit. The cause of the liver disease in these patients may be related to use of medications but the cause of the cerebrovascular disease in FMS patients is yet to be determined.

LEGAL ISSUES–THE DAUBERT STANDARD GOVERNING THE ADMISSIBILITY OF EXPERT TESTIMONY

The U.S. Supreme Court's opinion in Daubert v. Merrell Dow [1993] has given the judge the right to make an independent judicial assessment of the reliability of certain forms of expert testimony and to exclude testimony that he/she deems scientifically unacceptable. It was hoped that the new approach would end the current "battle of the experts" state of affairs. The original Daubert decision involved the claim that Bendectin caused birth defects. Even though the new judicial test was intended to clear the way to admission of novel scientific evidence with sound science [like DNA evidence], it has instead turned out to be a firestorm of controversy (Michael Finch, Professor of Law, Stetson University College of Law, 2004, personal communication).

The misuse of scientific evidence is certainly a serious problem. Even the FBI laboratory is under suspicion. In West Virginia, a serologist falsified test results in hundreds of cases over a ten-year period, resulting in the inappropriate sentencing of hundreds of defendants to lengthy prison terms. In Texas, a pathologist faked autopsy results, leading to as many as 20 death penalty verdicts. A police chemist elsewhere falsified reports and sent hundreds of innocent people to jail on rape charges. Most misuse of scientific evidence is pro-prosecution. The Daubert test has the potential to shed light on shoddy procedures, protocols, and proficiency testing. The risk from Daubert-related pre-trial decisions, however, is that relevant testimony will not be heard because it has been excluded on the basis of a judge's opinion. An even more egregious miscarriage of justice might occur if the judge is inadequately informed, misinformed, or biased against a point of view for reasons that are not readily apparent. For example, such biases could exclude testimony in support of a FMS patient's claim of injury contributing to their symptoms. As of 1999, 10 states, including Texas, have accepted Daubert, 14 states favor the alternative Frye Standard, and 12 states have their own standard. This leaves 14 states for which information on the subject is uncertain.

REFERENCES

1. Simons DG, Travell JG, Simons LS: Myofascial Pain and Dysfunction: The Trigger Point Manual, Volume 1. Upper Half of Body. Williams & Wilkins, Baltimore, 1999.

2. Travell JG, Simons DG: Myofascial Pain and Dysfunction: The Trigger Point Manual; Volume 2: Lower Half of Body. Williams & Wilkins, Baltimore, 1992.

3. Wolfe F, Smythe HA, Yunus MB, Bennett RM, Bombardier C, Goldenberg DL, Tugwell P, Campbell SM, Abeles M, Clark P, Fam AG, Farber SJ, Fiechtner JJ, Franklin CM, Gatter RA, Hamaty D, Lessard J, Lichtbroun AS, Masi AT, McCain GA, Reynolds WJ, Romano TJ, Russell IJ, Sheon RP: The American College of Rheumatology 1990 criteria for the classification of fibromyalgia. Arthritis Rheum 33: 160-172, 1990.

4. Wolfe F: Stop using the American College of Rheumatology criteria in the clinic. J Rheumatol 30(8): 1671-1672, 2003.

5. Jain AK, Carruthers BM, van de Sande MI, Barron SR, Donaldson CCS, Dunne JV, Gingrich E, Heffez DS, Leung FY-K, Malone DJ, Romano TJ, Russell IJ, Saul D, Seibel DG: Fibromyalgia syndrome: Canadian clinical working case definition, diagnostic and treatment protocols, a consensus document. J Musculoske Pain 11(4): 7-112, 2003.

6. Kersh BC, Bradley LA, Alarcon GS, Alberts KR, Sotolongo A, Martin MY, Aaron LA, Dewaal DF, Domino ML, Chaplin WF, Palardy NR, Cianfrini LR, Triana-Alexander M: Psychosocial and health status variables independently predict health care seeking in fibromyalgia. Arthritis Rheum 45: 362-371, 2001.

7. Aaron LA, Bradley LA, Alarcon GS, Alexander RW, Triana-Alexander M, Martin MY, Alberts KR: Psychiatric diagnoses in patients with fibromyalgia are related to health care-seeking behavior rather than to illness. Arthritis Rheum 39: 436-445, 1996.

8. Wilson RB, Gluck OS, Tesser JR, Rice JC, Meyer A, Bridges AJ: Antipolymer antibody reactivity in a subset of patients with fibromyalgia correlates with severity. J Rheumatol 26: 402-407, 1999.

9. Graven-Nielsen T, Aspegren KS, Henriksson KG, Bengtsson M, Sorensen J, Johnson A, Gerdle B, Arendt-Nielsen L: Ketamine reduces muscle pain, temporal summation, and referred pain in fibromyalgia patients. Pain 85: 483-491, 2000.

10. Giovengo SL, Russell IJ, Larson AA: Increased concentrations of nerve growth factor in cerebrospinal fluid of patients with fibromyalgia. J Rheumatol 26: 1564-1569, 1999.

11. Levy RI, Fredrickson DS: Diagnosis and management of hyperlipoproteinemia. Am J Cardiol 22(4): 576-583, 1968.

12. Caro XJ: Is there an immunologic component to the fibrositis syndrome? Rheum Dis Clin North Am 15: 169-186, 1989.

13. Gur A, Karakoc M, Nas K, Remzi, Cevik, Denli A, Wallace DJ: Cytokines and depression in cases with fibromyalgia. J Rheumatol 29(2): 358-361, 2002.

14. Wallace DJ, Linker-Israeli M, Hallegua D, Silverman S, Silver D, Weisman MH: Cytokines play an aetiopathogenetic role in fibromyalgia: A hypothesis and pilot study. Rheumatology 40: 743-749, 2001.

15. Torpy DJ, Papanicolaou DA, Lotsikas AJ, Wilder RL, Chrousos GP, Pillemer SR: Responses of the sympathetic nervous system and the hypothalamic-pituitary-adrenal axis to interleukin-6: A pilot study in fibromyalgia. Arthritis Rheum 43: 872-880, 2000.

16. Buskila D, Neumann L, Hazanov I, Carmi R: Familial aggregation in the fibromyalgia syndrome. Semin Arthritis Rheum 26: 605-611, 1996.

17. Pellegrino MJ, Waylonis GW, Sommer A: Familial occurrence of primary fibromyalgia. Arch Phys Med Rehabil 70: 61-63, 1989.

18. Buskila D, Neumann L, Hazanov I, Carmi R: Familial aggregation in the fibromyalgia syndrome. Semin Arthritis Rheum 26: 605-611, 1996.

19. Yunus MB, Khan MA, Rawlings KK, Green JR, Olson JM, Shah S: Genetic linkage analysis of multicase families with fibromyalgia syndrome. J Rheumatol 26: 408-412, 1999.

20. Iyengar SK, Arnold LM, Khan MA, Russell IJ, Yunus MB, Hess E, Humphrey J, Russo K, Dudek DM, Olson JM: Genetic Linkage of Fibromyalgia Syndrome to the Serotonin Receptor 2A Region on Chromosome 13 and the HLA Region on Chromosome 6. Genes Immunity, 2005 (in press).

21. Gursoy S, Erdal E, Herken H, Madenci E, Alasehirli B, Erdal N: Significance of catechol-O-methyltransferase gene polymorphism in fibromyalgia syndrome. Rheumatol Int 23(3): 104-107, 2003.

22. Zubieta JK, Heitzeg MM, Smith YR, Bueller JA, Xu K, Xu Y: COMT val158-met genotype affects mu-opioid neurotransmitter responses to a pain stressor. Science 299(5610): 1240-1243, 2003.

23. Galeotti N, Ghelardini C, Zippi M, Cel Bene E, Beneforti E, Bartonini A: A Reduced Functionality of Gi Proteins as a Possible Cause of Fibromyalgia. J Rheumatol 28: 2298-2304, 2001.

24. Maekawa K, Twe C, Lotaif A, Chiappelli F, Clark GT: Function of beta-adrenergic receptors on mononuclear cells in female patients with fibromyalgia. J Rheumatol 30: 364-368, 2003.

25. Bennett RM, Clark SR, Campbell SM, Burckhardt CS: Low levels of somatomedin C in patients with the fibromyalgia syndrome. A possible link between sleep and muscle pain. Arthritis Rheum 35: 1113-1116, 1992.

26. Bennett RM, Clark SC, Walczyk J: A randomized, double-blind, placebo-controlled study of growth hormone in the treatment of fibromyalgia. Am J Med 104: 227-231, 1998.

27. Paiva ES, Deodhar A, Jones KD, Bennett RM: Impaired growth hormone secretion in fibromyalgia patients: Evidence for augmented hypothalamic somatostatin tone. Arthritis Rheum 46(5): 1344-1350, 2002.

28. Meyer HP, Van der Westhuizen FD: Impact of spinal surgery in patients with fibromyalgia syndrome and backpain. J Musculoske Pain 12(suppl#9): 61, 2004.

29. Dreyer L, Kendall SA, Winther JF, Mellemkjaer L, Danneskiold-Samsoe B, Bliddal H: Increased suicide, liver disease, and cerebrovascular disease mortality in a cohort of Danish patients with fibromyalgia. J Musculoske Pain 12(Suppl#9): 49, 2004.

Diagnostic Criteria and Differential Diagnosis of the Fibromyalgia Syndrome

Robert M. Bennett

SUMMARY. Objectives: The goals of this presentation are to review the American College of Rheumatology [ACR] research classification criteria for the fibromyalgia syndrome [FMS] and to show how they facilitate the differential diagnosis of pain in a variety of clinical presentations.

Findings: The ACR criteria were developed directly from a research validation study and apply best to that setting. In lieu of a better resource, these criteria have been applied to community clinical practice as well. The design of the ACR Criteria study is outlined. The results show how the ACR Criteria directly follow the study findings. In patients with chronic widespread pain, the presence of 11 of 18 anatomically defined tender points [TePs] sufficiently sensitized to be painful when stimulated by four kilograms of digital pressure identified FMS irrespective of concomitant conditions, including conditions with the potential to cause pain. The ACR criteria depend only on pain, so they do not take into consideration other common features of FMS, such as insomnia, visceral syndromes, headache, or affective symptoms. The ACR Criteria definition allows the concomitant diagnosis of FMS in patients known to have painful rheumatic, neurological, infectious, neoplastic, inherited, and acquired disorders.

Conclusions: The ACR criteria for FMS were developed to facilitate research regarding this common painful condition, but have been applied to community clinical care as well. These criteria distinguish FMS from other painful disorders and disclose overlapping diagnoses. *[Article copies available for a fee from The Haworth Document Delivery Service: 1-800-HAWORTH. E-mail address: <docdelivery@haworthpress.com> Website: <http://www.HaworthPress.com> © 2004 by The Haworth Press, Inc. All rights reserved.]*

KEYWORDS. Fibromyalgia syndrome, classification criteria, diagnostic criteria, differential diagnosis

THE 1990 AMERICAN COLLEGE OF RHEUMATOLOGY CLASSIFICATION CRITERIA

The American College of Rheumatology [ACR] 1990 criteria for the classification of Fibromyalgia Syndrome [FMS] are currently a sine qua non for identifying FMS subjects in scientific research protocols. It is sometimes forgotten that these criteria were intended for purposes of classification but are now extensively used for diagnostic purposes. Indeed, in the discussion from the 1990 criteria paper it was noted that "the sensitivity of the criteria suggests that they may be useful for diagnosis as well as classification" (1).

I suspect that most clinicians and researchers have not carefully read/re-read the 1990 ACR

Robert M. Bennett, MD, FRCP, is Professor of Medicine, Oregon Health and Science University, Portland, OR, USA.

[Haworth co-indexing entry note]: "Diagnostic Criteria and Differential Diagnosis of the Fibromyalgia Syndrome." Bennett, Robert M. Co-published simultaneously in *Journal of Musculoskeletal Pain* [The Haworth Medical Press, an imprint of The Haworth Press, Inc.] Vol. 12, No. 3/4, 2004, pp. 59-64; and: *Soft Tissue Pain Syndromes: Clinical Diagnosis and Pathogenesis* [ed: Dieter E. Pongratz, Siegfried Mense, and Michael Spaeth] The Haworth Medical Press, an imprint of The Haworth Press, Inc., 2004, pp. 59-64. Single or multiple copies of this article are available for a fee from The Haworth Document Delivery Service [1-800-HAWORTH, 9:00 a.m. - 5:00 p.m. [EST]. E-mail address: docdelivery@haworthpress.com].

criteria for some time. It is therefore appropriate to list the salient points of this frequently quoted paper.

Study Design

1. A multicenter study conducted in 16 separate centers in the United States and Canada.
2. The study was conducted on 293 subjects considered to have FMS by the principal investigator and 265 control patients. These controls were made up of patients with neck and low back pain syndromes, tendinitis, post-traumatic pain, lupus, rheumatoid arthritis, and osteoarthritis.
3. Each investigator was asked to provide 10 patients with primary FMS, 10 patients with secondary or concomitant FMS and 20 age and sex matched pain controls.
4. Prior to performing the study investigator training sessions were held to standardize the methodology for tender point palpation and dolorimetry.
5. Tender point examinations were conducted by investigators blinded to preliminary diagnoses and symptomatic questionnaires.
6. Twenty-four tender point locations and six "control" locations were evaluated by palpation.
7. Six tender point locations and three "control" were assessed by dolorimetry.
8. Twenty-seven symptoms related to pain, modulating factors, and features considered to be common in FMS [e.g., sleep disturbance, fatigue, irritable bowel, etc.] were recorded.

Study Results

1. The mean age all subjects was 48. Subjects with secondary/concomitant FMS were significantly older [7.2 years] than subjects with primary FMS.
2. Eighty-eight percent of the subjects were female.
3. Widespread pain was reported in 97 percent of FMS subjects and 70 percent of pain controls.

4. Non-pain symptoms such as fatigue, sleep disturbance, and morning stiffness were found in 73-85 percent of FMS subjects and 22-40 percent of controls.
5. There was no significant difference between primary FMS secondary/concomitant FMS subjects as regards pain characteristics and tender points.
6. Fibromyalgia subjects had a mean tender point count of 19.3 [out of the 24 sites examined] compared to 7.7 in controls.
7. Tender points were the most powerful discriminate between FMS subjects and controls.
8. An operator-receiver curve analysis indicated that the best separation between FMS subjects and controls occurred at the 13th tender point [defined as mild or greater pain]. Subsequently three paired tender point locations [lateral pectoral at the level of the fourth rib in the anterior axillary line, paraspinous muscles just lateral to the midline at the level of the scapula, and the medial epicondyle] were discarded due to a low discriminatory power. Thus the final criteria recommended an examination of nine paired tender points with a classification cutoff at 11 or more tender points.
9. The combination of widespread pain [defined as axial plus three or more quadrants] and the finding of moderate or greater tenderness in ≥ 11 of 18 tender points yielded a diagnostic sensitivity of 88.4 percent and a specificity of 81.1 percent.
10. The inclusion of symptoms such as sleep disturbance, fatigue, and morning stiffness in various combinations with widespread pain and ≥ 11 of 18 tender points reduced the diagnostic sensitivity and specificity.
11. Primary and secondary/concomitant FMS were indistinguishable, using the study variables, and the committee suggested abolishing the distinction between primary and secondary/concomitant FMS.

The final classification criteria were:

1. *History of widespread pain*

   Pain is considered widespread when all of the following are present: pain in the left side of the body, pain in the right side of the body, pain above the waist, and pain below the waist. In addition, axial skeletal pain [cervical spine or anterior chest or thoracic spine or low back] must be present. In this definition, shoulder and buttock pain is considered as pain for each involved side. "Low back" pain is considered lower segment pain.

2. *Pain in 11 of 18 tender point sites on digital palpation*

   Pain, on digital palpation, must be present in at least 11 of the following 18 sites:

   Occiput: Bilateral, at the suboccipital muscle insertions.

   Low cervical: bilateral, at the anterior aspects of the intertransverse spaces at C5-C7.

   Trapezius: bilateral, at the midpoint of the upper border.

   Supraspinatus: bilateral, at origins, above the scapula spine near the medial border.

   Second rib: bilateral, at the second costochondral junctions, just lateral to the junctions on upper surfaces.

   Lateral epicondyle: bilateral, 2 cm distal to the epicondyles.

   Gluteal: bilateral, in upper outer quadrants of buttocks in anterior fold of muscle.

   Greater trochanter: bilateral, posterior to the trochanteric prominence.

   Knee: bilateral, at the medial fat pad proximal to the joint line.

   Digital palpation should be performed with an approximate force of 4 kg. For a tender point to be considered "positive" the subject must state that the palpation was painful. "Tender" is not to be considered "painful."

Classification

For classification purposes, patients will be said to have FMS if both criteria are satisfied. Widespread pain must have been present for at least three months. The presence of a second clinical disorder does not exclude the diagnosis of FMS.

PROBLEMS WITH THE 1990 AMERICAN COLLEGE OF RHEUMATOLOGY CRITERIA

As is the case with most other rheumatological criteria, the 1990 ACR criteria are based on "circular reasoning" in that those subjects entered into the study as having FMS were defined by the local expert as having that diagnosis. This is an inevitable result of not having a gold standard "diagnostic test" for FMS. However, this "best shot" approach to establishing diagnostic criteria is widely used in many medical disorders that lack a gold standard [e.g., all psychiatric disorders, rheumatoid arthritis, systemic lupus erythematosus, vascular headaches, irritable bowel syndrome, vasculitic disorders, chronic fatigue syndrome, restless leg syndrome, etc.].

The relevance of tender points in the diagnosis of FMS has subsequently been a topic for opinion and debate. Epidemiological studies examining the prevalence of widespread pain [WSP] as defined in the ACR criteria [i.e., pain in three out of four quadrants of the body] found WSP to be some four times more prevalent than ACR criteria defined FMS (2-4) and that pain distribution is a continuum, with a positive correlation to the number of tender points and psychological distress (5-7). Viewed from this perspective FMS can be viewed as being at the extreme end of the pain spectrum, and analogies have been made with the other disease-spectrum disorders such as those involving blood pressure and cholesterol.

However, in the multicenter study on which the 1990 ACR criteria are based some 70 percent of pain controls fulfilled the definition of WSP and the most discriminatory feature between FMS patients and other pain disorders was the finding of tender points above and below the waist. White et al. have reaffirmed the usefulness of tender points in an epidemiological study of subjects with WSP (8).

It is sometimes forgotten, or even unrecognized, that FMS patients usually have multiple tender points other than those specified by the 1990 ACR criteria. Indeed, the study upon which the 1990 ACR criteria were based initially evaluated 24 tender point locations. Although the term "tender point" is usually used specifically when describing painful areas in relation to a diagnosis of FMS, it is my clinical experience that there is no clinical difference between FMS tender points and myofascial trigger points. Although the FMS tender points in the anterior neck, anterior chest and medial knee are described in non-muscle terms [i.e., the anterior aspects of the intertransverse spaces at C5-C7, the second costochondral junctions just lateral to the junctions on upper surfaces, and the medial fat pad proximal to the joint line, respectively], these locations can also be described in terms of myofascial trigger points that are located at the lower attachment of the sternocleidomastoid muscle to the clavicle, the medial portion of the pectoralis minor muscle and the lower end of the vastus medialis muscle, respectively. If this impression is correct there are at least five important corollaries: 1. in that numerous myofascial trigger point locations have been identified in the non-FMS literature (9-11), the 18 tender locations used in the current FMS criteria represent a sampling of approximately three percent of the total possible tender points; 2. the finding of 10 or less tender points in some patients, who otherwise have the classical features of FMS, is an inevitable result of a sampling error; 3. FMS needs to be differentiated from widespread myofascial pain, and it is proposed that the crucial difference is development of central sensitization and the "systemic" features of nonrestorative sleep, fatigue, and subtle neuroendocrine dysfunction; 4. myofascial trigger points are potentially important peripheral pain generators in driving the process of central sensitization; and 5. FMS patients' perception of pain as arising from muscle probably has a physiological basis in terms of central sensitization causing an "increased volume" of nociceptive impulses arising from myofascial trigger points.

REVISED CRITERIA

The 1990 ACR classification criteria were a major turning point for enabling scientific studies investigating the epidemiology, clinical characteristics, and pathophysiological aberrations in patients with FMS to be conducted on a uniform population of subjects. As a clinician, I'm constantly impressed with the applicability and usefulness of these criteria in the care of rheumatology patients. In the decade prior to 1990 there were 210 articles referring to FMS in either the title or abstract that were cited in the National Library of Medicine database, whereas in the following decade 2,260 articles on FMS were cited. However, clinical investigators are always eager to revise and redefine diagnostic criteria and it is inevitable that the 1990 ACR criteria will eventually be revisited as scientific advances substantiate objective differences between patients with FMS and healthy individuals. As the present time there is persuasive evidence that FMS could be redefined in terms of widespread central sensitization (12). If this were generally agreed upon an objective test of central sensitization could potentially replace the current examination of tender points. There is currently no agreement as to the technology for such an evaluation. Of the three main methods that are currently used to demonstrate abnormal sensory processing in FMS patients [i.e., the demonstration of increased temporal summation to cutaneous heat (13) or muscle stimulation (14), the functional magnetic resonance imaging response to experimental pain (15,16), and the nociceptive flexion reflex (8083,8457)], the nociceptive flexion reflex is the most likely to gain widespread acceptance as it employs the same apparatus as is used in standard electromyogram/NCV testing.

DIFFERENTIAL DIAGNOSIS

The 1990 ACR classification criteria imply that FMS is not a diagnosis of exclusion and no distinction is made between primary and secondary/concomitant FMS. This is an important concept as there is often a tendency to consider a diagnosis of FMS only after all other possibilities have been excluded. This "negative" approach to diagnosis often leads to unnecessary and sometimes costly investigations. A critical concept in understanding FMS is that it often arises as a concomitant problem in many other disorders, particularly those that are associated with pain [see Table 1].

As many of these disorders are potential peripheral pain generators, their accurate diagnosis and management is critical to the comprehensive treatment of FMS patients (36,37). With the increasing acceptance of FMS as a common diagnosis, rheumatologists are increasingly seeing patients diagnosed as having FMS who have other diagnoses (38). In most cases the patient does in fact have FMS, but the referring practitioner has missed another rheumatic problem that is often relevant to effective management. Commonly associated diagnoses that are often overlooked include musculoskeletal pain problems such as bursitis/tendinitis, compression neuropathies and myofascial pain syndromes, hypermobility syndrome and rheumatic disorders such as osteoarthritis, early rheumatoid arthritis, early ankylosing spondylitis, polymyalgia rheumatica, and lupus. Occasionally endocrine disorders such as hypothyroidism and early acromegaly may present with symptoms of widespread pain. Osteomalacia, especially when it presents with a painful myopathy, is easily mistaken for FMS and should be considered in all elderly patients, as well as those living in areas with little sunlight and patients with eating disorders or restricted diets.

TABLE 1

Low back pain	(17)
Post whiplash pain	(18)
Injuries	(19)
Hypermobility syndrome	(20)
Sickle cell disease	(21)
Rheumatoid arthritis	(22)
Systemic lupus erythematosus	(23)
Sjogren's syndrome	(24)
Small intestine bacterial overgrowth	(25)
Crohn's disease	(26)
Parvovirus infections	(27)
HIV infection	(28)
Familial Mediterranean fever	(29)
Hepatitis C	(30)
Lyme disease	(31)
Endometriosis	(32)
Growing pains	(33)
Hereditary myopathies	(34)
Myofascial pain	(35)

REFERENCES

1. Wolfe F, Smythe HA, Yunus MB, Bennett RM, Bombardier C, Goldenberg DL, Tugwell P, Campbell SM, Abeles M, Clark P, Fam AG, Farber SJ, Fiechtner JJ, Franklin CM, Gatter RA, Hamaty D, Lessard J, Lichtbroun AS, Masi AT, McCain GA, Reynolds WJ, Romano TJ, Russell IJ, Sheon R. The American College of Rheumatology 1990 criteria for the classification of fibromyalgia: Report of the Multicenter Criteria Committee. Arth Rheum 33:160-172, 1990.

2. MacFarlane GJ. Generalized pain, fibromyalgia and regional pain: An epidemiological view. Baillieres Best Pract Res Clin Rheumatol 13(3):403-414, 1999.

3. Wolfe F, Cathey MA. The epidemiology of tender points: A prospective study of 1520 patients. J Rheumatol 12:1164-1168, 1985.

4. Wolfe F, Ross K, Anderson J, Russell IJ, Hebert L. The prevalence and characteristics of fibromyalgia in the general population. Arth Rheum 38:19-28, 1995.

5. McBeth J, MacFarlane GJ, Benjamin S, Morris S, Silman AJ. The association between tender points, psychological distress, and adverse childhood experiences: A community-based study. Arthritis Rheum 42(7):1397-1404, 1999.

6. Giesecke T, Williams DA, Harris RE, Cupps TR, Tian X, Tian TX, Gracely RH, Clauw DJ. Subgrouping of fibromyalgia patients on the basis of pressure-pain thresholds and psychological factors. Arthritis Rheum 48(10):2916-2922, 2003.

7. Clauw DJ, Crofford LJ. Chronic widespread pain and fibromyalgia: What we know, and what we need to know. Best Pract Res Clin Rheumatol 17(4):685-701, 2003.

8. White KP, Harth M, Speechley M, Ostbye T. A general population study of fibromyalgia tender points in noninstitutionalized adults with chronic widespread pain. J Rheumatol 27(11):2677-2682, 2000.

9. Travell JG, Simons DG. Myofascial pain and dysfunction: The trigger point manual. Baltimore: Williams & Wilkins, 1983.

10. Travell J, Simons D. Myofascial Pain and Dysfunction: The trigger point manual, Volume 2. Baltimore: Williams & Wilkins, 1992.

11. Gerwin RD. Classification, epidemiology, and natural history of myofascial pain syndrome. Curr Pain Headache Rep 5(5):412-420, 2001.

12. Staud R. Evidence of involvement of central neural mechanisms in generating fibromyalgia pain. Curr Rheumatol Rep 4(4):299-305, 2002.

13. Staud R, Vierck CJ, Cannon RL, Mauderli AP, Price DD. Abnormal sensitization and temporal summation of second pain (wind-up) in patients with fibromyalgia syndrome. Pain 91(1-2):165-175, 2001.

14. Staud R, Cannon RC, Mauderli AP, Robinson ME, Price DD, Vierck CJ. Temporal summation of pain from mechanical stimulation of muscle tissue in normal controls and subjects with fibromyalgia syndrome. Pain 102(1-2):87-95, 2003.

15. Gracely RH, Petzke F, Wolf JM, Clauw DJ. Functional magnetic resonance imaging evidence of augmented pain processing in fibromyalgia. Arthritis Rheum 46(5):1333-1343, 2002.

16. Cook DB, Lange G, Ciccone DS, Liu WC, Steffener J, Natelson BH. Functional imaging of pain in patients with primary fibromyalgia. J Rheumatol 31(2): 364-378, 2004.

17. Lapossy E, Maleitzke R, Hrycaj P, Mennet W, Muller W. The frequency of transition of chronic low back pain to fibromyalgia. Scand J Rheumatol 24:29-33, 1995.

18. Buskila D, Neumann L, Vaisberg G, Alkalay D, Wolfe F. Increased rates of fibromyalgia following cervical spine injury. A controlled study of 161 cases of traumatic injury. Arthritis Rheum 40:446-452, 1997.

19. Al Allaf AW, Dunbar KL, Hallum NS, Nosratzadeh B, Templeton KD, Pullar T. A case-control study examining the role of physical trauma in the onset of fibromyalgia syndrome. Rheumatology (Oxford) 41(4):450-453, 2002.

20. Goldman JA. Fibromyalgia and hypermobility. J Rheumatol 28(4):920-921, 2001.

21. Schlesinger N. Clues to pathogenesis of fibromyalgia in patients with sickle cell disease. J Rheumatol 31(3):598-600, 2004.

22. Naranjo A, Ojeda S, Francisco F, Erausquin C, Rua-Figueroa I, Rodriguez-Lozano C. Fibromyalgia in patients with rheumatoid arthritis is associated with higher scores of disability. Ann Rheum Dis 61(7):660-661, 2002.

23. Grafe A, Wollina U, Tebbe B, Sprott H, Uhlemann C, Hein G. Fibromyalgia in lupus erythematosus. Acta Derm Venereol 79(1):62-64, 1999.

24. Ostuni P, Botsios C, Sfriso P, Punzi L, Chieco-Bianchi F, Semerano L et al. Fibromyalgia in Italian patients with primary Sjogren's syndrome. Joint Bone Spine 69(1):51-57, 2002.

25. Pimentel M, Wallace D, Hallegua D, Chow E, Kong Y, Park S et al. A link between irritable bowel syndrome and fibromyalgia may be related to findings on lactulose breath testing. Ann Rheum Dis 63(4): 450-452, 2004.

26. Buskila D, Odes LR, Neumann L, Odes HS. Fibromyalgia in inflammatory bowel disease. J Rheumatol 26(5):1167-1171, 1999.

27. Leventhal LJ, Naides SJ, Freundlich B. Fibromyalgia and parvovirus infection. Arth Rheum 34: 1319-1324, 1991.

28. Simms RW, Ferrante N, Craven DE. High prevalence of fibromyalgia syndrome (FMS) in human immunodeficiency virus type 1 (HIV) infected patients with polyarthralgia. Arth Rheum 33(9):S136, 1990.

29. Langevitz P, Buskila D, Finkelstein R, Zaks N, Neuman L, Sukenik S et al. Fibromyalgia in familial Mediterranean fever. J Rheumatol 21:1335-1337, 1994.

30. Barkhuizen A, Schoeplin GS, Bennett RM. Fibromyalgia: A prominent feature in patients with musculoskeletal problems in chronic hepatitis C: A report of 12 patients. J Clinical Rheumatology 2:180-184, 1996.

31. Dinerman H, Steere AC. Fibromyalgia following Lyme disease: Association with neurologic involvement and lack of response to antibiotic therapy. Arth Rheum 33(9):S136, 1990.

32. Bajaj P, Bajaj P, Madsen H, Arendt-Nielsen L. Endometriosis is associated with central sensitization: A psychophysical controlled study. J Pain 4(7):372-380, 2003.

33. Hashkes PJ, Friedland O, Jaber L, Cohen HA, Wolach B, Uziel Y. Decreased pain threshold in children with growing pains. J Rheumatol 31(3):610-613, 2004.

34. Gerra G, Zaimovic A, Giucastro G, Folli F, Maestri D, Tessoni A, Avanzini P, Caccavari R, Bernasconi S, Brambilla F. Neurotransmitter-hormonal responses to psychological stress in peripubertal subjects: Relationship to aggressive behavior. Life Sci 62(7):617-625, 1998.

35. Meyer HP. Myofascial pain syndrome and its suggested role in the pathogenesis and treatment of fibromyalgia syndrome. Curr Pain Headache Rep 6(4): 274-283, 2002.

36. Daoud KF, Barkhuizen A. Rheumatic mimics and selected triggers of fibromyalgia. Curr Pain Headache Rep 6(4):284-288, 2002.

37. Borg-Stein J. Management of peripheral pain generators in fibromyalgia. Rheum Dis Clin North Am 28(2):305-317, 2002.

38. Fitzcharles MA, Boulos P. Inaccuracy in the diagnosis of fibromyalgia syndrome: Analysis of referrals. Rheumatology (Oxford) 42(2):263-267, 2003.

Fibromyalgia:
Novel Therapeutic Aspects

Carol S. Burckhardt

SUMMARY. Objectives: This paper focuses on nonpharmacologic approaches to fibromyalgia treatment. Descriptions of the most well researched strategies, such as exercise, cognitive-behavioral therapy, and multidisciplinary treatment using multiple treatment components, along with novel treatments for which evidence is beginning to emerge, are compared and evaluated.

Findings: Evidence for the pain reduction benefits of moderate intensity exercise is strong. Both cognitive-behavioral therapy as a stand-alone treatment and multicomponent strategies that incorporate exercise and cognitive-behavioral or education strategies have significant benefits to patients mainly in enhanced self-efficacy and physical capacity and decreased pain. Novel therapies such as acupuncture, biofeedback, balneotherapy, therapeutic massage, movement therapy, vegetarian diets and supplements, and magnets all demonstrate therapeutic benefits in small clinical trials. There is some evidence that discernible characteristics may differentiate responders from nonresponders to many therapies.

Conclusions: Overall, there is moderate to strong evidence of the effectiveness of some nonpharmacologic approaches to fibromyalgia treatment. Novel treatments from a wide group of practitioners and health perspectives are beginning to emerge as legitimate strategies. An individualized approach that incorporates patient's abilities, preferences, physical and psychological characteristics is critical to the success of treatment. *[Article copies available for a fee from The Haworth Document Delivery Service: 1-800-HAWORTH. E-mail address: <docdelivery@haworthpress.com> Website: <http://www.HaworthPress.com> © 2004 by The Haworth Press, Inc. All rights reserved.]*

KEYWORDS. Fibromyalgia, treatment, novel approaches, review

Symptom management is the principal treatment currently available to fibromyalgia syndrome [FMS] patients. Because patients typically present with complex symptoms and comorbid conditions, they can not be expected to respond to single medications or strategies. Multiple strategies that include medications, physical, cognitive, behavioral, and educational aspects, are essential to comprehensive and effective treatment. Additionally, novel therapies that come from complementary and alternative medicine [CAM] perspectives are beginning to emerge as viable and effective treatments.

Typically, therapeutic approaches in FMS treatment encompass two types of strategies, those that are largely self-managed, such as cognitive coping skills, exercise, and healthful behaviors, and those that are provided by prac-

Carol S. Burckhardt, RN, PhD, is Professor of Nursing and Assistant Professor of Medicine [Research], School of Nursing–SN ORD, Oregon Health & Science University, 3181 SW Sam Jackson Park Road, Portland, OR 97239 USA.

[Haworth co-indexing entry note]: "Fibromyalgia: Novel Therapeutic Aspects." Burckhardt. Carol S. Co-published simultaneously in *Journal of Musculoskeletal Pain* [The Haworth Medical Press, an imprint of The Haworth Press, Inc.] Vol. 12, No. 3/4, 2004, pp. 65-72; and: *Soft Tissue Pain Syndromes: Clinical Diagnosis and Pathogenesis* [ed: Dieter E. Pongratz, Siegfried Mense, and Michael Spaeth] The Haworth Medical Press, an imprint of The Haworth Press, Inc., 2004, pp. 65-72. Single or multiple copies of this article are available for a fee from The Haworth Document Delivery Service [1-800-HAWORTH, 9:00 a.m. - 5:00 p.m. [EST]. E-mail address: docdelivery@haworthpress.com].

Available online at http://www.haworthpress.com/web/JMP
© 2004 by The Haworth Press, Inc. All rights reserved.
doi:10.1300/J094v12n03_10

titioners, such as medication management and physical therapy. Long-term success of any therapeutic regimen depends on patients' ongoing, self-motivation to monitor their symptoms, practice the skills they have been taught, and access professionals for expert advice and treatment at appropriate times. If patients are to carry out this work, they and their health care providers need evidence-based knowledge regarding the efficacy of treatment strategies, reliable and valid methods of measuring symptom change, procedures for implementing strategies, and individualized treatment plans.

A number of FMS treatment reviews have been published in recent years including evaluations of exercise (1,2), cognitive-behavioral therapy [CBT] (3), and patient education (4). These strategy-specific reviews along with evaluations of multidisciplinary management and rehabilitation (5,6), physical therapy (7), as well as general reviews (8-10), all suggest with varying level of confidence and caution, that some treatments improve functioning and decrease FMS symptoms.

This paper briefly summarizes the evidence base for four of the most widely accepted approaches to treatment of FMS [patient education, CBT, exercise, and multicomponent programs]. Then it focuses on newer, more unique approaches to treatment and evaluates those that have, at present, some evidence in the scientific literature. Finally, some evidence for differential responses to treatment are presented and methods for deriving maximal benefit from treatment strategies are suggested.

PATIENT EDUCATION, COGNITIVE-BEHAVIORAL THERAPY, EXERCISE, AND MULTICOMPONENT STRATEGIES

Patient Education

Four randomized controlled trials [RCTs] with FMS patients have focused specifically on patient education as the experimental treatment and compared the experimental group to a wait-list control group (11-14). The treatments were described as information-focused education given in group format using lectures, written materials, group discussions, and demonstra-

tions. Length of the education treatment ranged from six-12 weeks with one study having follow-up monthly sessions for 10 months (13). Only two (11,13) found significant changes on any outcome at the end of the study. The education groups were significantly better than the control groups on self-efficacy and quality of life in the first study and had less helplessness in the latter. These results suggest that group education alone is not sufficient to change symptoms.

Cognitive-Behavioral Therapy

Cognitive-behavioral therapy is a generic term that incorporates a wide-range of treatment modalities [e.g., stress management, distraction, relaxation, cognitive restructuring] all of which are designed to enhance coping, facilitate self-management, and improve function. Cognitive-behavioral therapy as a stand-alone treatment has produced significant short-term effects on pain severity, pain coping, self-efficacy, and functional status in four RCTs when compared to treatment as usual or no treatment control groups (14-17). The number of sessions ranged from six to 20. Basic elements of stress reduction and pain management skills were emphasized in three trials while one trial emphasized improvement in physical functioning (17).

Two studies that used cognitive-behavioral intervention as the experimental treatment and patient education as the attention control found that subjects in the patient education group changed as much on the outcome variables as the CBT experimental group subjects (16,18). In both of these trials, the attention control was a well-planned educational program and not a sham or placebo treatment. The research evidence for CBT can be rated moderate at this point due to the very consistent findings from multiple RCTs.

Exercise

A Cochrane review has reported strong evidence from four high quality RCTs that aerobic exercise produces increased cardiovascular fitness, pain pressure thresholds, global well-being, and self-efficacy for functioning in patients with FMS (1). Two high quality muscle strength studies (19,20), one of which used stretching as a control condition, found significant improvement in muscle strength, depression, fatigue, and pain.

Although the evidence base for the cardiovascular benefits of aerobic exercise is strong, researchers have noted that high intensity aerobic exercise may be difficult, if not impossible, for many patients with FMS. Some have recently suggested that patients with FMS might benefit from lower intensity exercise and adhere to an exercise regimen that is graded and individualized. Evidence from a study of low intensity pool-based aerobic exercise indicated that such an approach was beneficial (21). Another study found clear evidence that graded aerobic exercise that allowed subjects to increase their exercise as tolerated over a 12 week period resulted in significant increases in duration and intensity as well as significant positive changes in self-rated global impression and decreases in tender points (22).

Multicomponent Strategies

A number of studies provide evidence for the efficacy of treatment by multidisciplinary teams using multicomponent strategies for people with FMS. Of seven RCTs that combined exercise with patient education and/or CBT, six resulted in significant improvements for the experimental treatment group on one or more outcomes at the end of treatment (11,12,21,23-26). Five of these trials have been rated as moderate or high quality and all have very consistent findings of treatment efficacy.

Treatment length ranged from six to 24 weeks. Self-efficacy was significantly enhanced in the treated groups. The Fibromyalgia Impact Questionnaire [FIQ] total score, a measure of overall FMS impact, was significantly decreased in only one study at the end of the RCT but showed significant decrease in three studies at three to six month follow-up. Pain was significantly decreased in four trials. Four of five RCTs that used a no treatment or wait list control group offered consistent evidence of the superiority of a multicomponent approach. One study that used a relaxation attention control did not show differences at end of treatment (26) while the other supported the multicomponent approach when compared to an attention control education program (24).

Unlike the single strategy approaches, a number of uncontrolled multicomponent studies have been completed over the past 10 years. Although the weaknesses of single group trials are well known, four studies with follow-up data (27-30) provide consistent evidence of positive changes in pain and FMS impact at the end of treatment that were maintained six to 30 months post-treatment. Thus, the research-based evidence for multicomponent trials at present can be considered moderate to strong because of the consistent evidence from multiple trials.

NOVEL THERAPEUTIC ASPECTS

For purposes of this paper, novel therapeutic aspects are defined as therapies that come from CAM perspectives and/or have few research studies that currently support their use in FMS treatment. The majority of these novel approaches require the ongoing services of experts with specialized training, are, for the most part, accessed outside the mainstream health care system and may add substantial out-of-pocket costs for the person with FMS. Consequently, if health care providers recommend them, patients need to know what benefit they might expect. Reviews of CAM therapies for FMS have been published recently (31-33).

Acupuncture

Acupuncture is a well-known and increasingly well-accepted form of treatment for painful musculoskeletal problems. A review of acupuncture treatment in FMS (34) concluded that the one high-quality RCT in the extant literature (35) provided evidence that acupuncture is more effective than sham acupuncture for relieving pain, increasing pain thresholds, and decreasing morning stiffness. A number of small studies have consistently confirmed these findings. Berman and colleagues caution, however, that exacerbations of FMS pain can occur with acupuncture treatment perhaps due to pain amplification secondary to needle trauma. In the high-quality study 15 percent of the subjects withdrew because of increased pain. This possibility should be considered when recommending acupuncture to patients with FMS.

Biofeedback

A study of electromyography-biofeedback training in FMS patients concluded that nine of 15 subjects benefited significantly from the treatment and that the effects lasted for up to six months (36). Since this early study, three studies of biofeedback alone and one combining exercise and biofeedback have been published. One found that electromyography-biofeedback had significant positive effects on pain, vitality, and mental health in a group of patients who had been classified as either psychologically normal or abnormal (37). Two others found no significant evidence that biofeedback alone was effective in changing symptoms (24,38). The Buckelew study found that biofeedback was more effective when combined with an exercise treatment. Thus the evidence for biofeedback is mixed at this point.

Balneotherapy

Balneotherapy, a general term for therapeutic bathing, and medicinal baths have been studied in Israel and Europe. One Israeli RCT (39) concluded that 10 days of sulfur baths resulted in significantly decreased tender points and visual analog scale pain scores in the treated group. An RCT from Turkey (40) found significant decreases in the number of tender points, pain, depression, and FIQ total scores in the group that was treated with 15-20-minute sessions of bathing in 36-degree water over a three week period. Improvements were still significant six months later. An Austrian RCT compared whirlpool baths with plain water to water containing either valerian or pine oil in a sample of 39 patients with FMS. The valerian treated group had significantly improved well being, sleep, and number of tender points while the group treated with plain water had reduced pain intensity (41). In a recent 12-week, randomized, comparison study of pool-based exercise and balneotherapy (42), both groups improved significantly on FIQ total score, pain, fatigue, stiffness, sleep, number of tender points, and global evaluation. These variables were also significantly improved from baseline at a 24-week follow-up. The evidence for balneotherapy is moderate with consistent results from multiple RCTs.

Therapeutic Massage

Three small RCTs of therapeutic massage have been published within the past five years. A Swedish study (43), using classical massage techniques for 15 sessions over 10 weeks found significant differences in current pain and FIQ total scores between the treatment and control group at the end of treatment. Treatment compliance in this study was high with only two subjects completing fewer than all 15 treatments and only four dropping out, all for reasons unrelated to the treatment. A Turkish study of classical massage compared to mobilization techniques found that subjects in both groups improved significantly in the number of trigger points and neck pain (44). An American study, which suffered a 53 percent dropout rate, showed no significant effects of massage when compared to standard care (45). Evidence from the two RCTs with low dropout rates is promising for short-term positive effects.

Movement Therapies

Movement therapies are defined here as physical actions that are intended to make the person more aware of the body and/or increase internal energy. They are different from exercise in that no attempt is made to increase aerobic capacity. Two RCTs, one of Qigong and meditation (46) and the other of two body awareness therapies (47), suggest that these therapies may be of some benefit. Reductions in pain, depression, FIQ total score as well as increases in self-efficacy, pain control, and global health were noted at the end of the trials and maintenance of changes at six month follow-up was demonstrated. Small pilot studies of Feldenkrais (48), T'ai Chi (49), and a multi-component trial of education, relaxation, and Qigong (50) contributed further evidence that movement therapies can benefit FMS patients by decreasing symptom impact and increasing function.

Diet and Supplements

In two open controlled diet trials, one of which compared diet to amitriptyline, a vegetarian diet for six weeks resulted in improved pain scores in the diet group while pain, fatigue, insomnia, and tender point counts all improved significantly in the amitriptyline group (51). The other, a strict vegan diet found that the vegan group was significantly improved on joint stiffness, sleep quality, pain, general health, and body mass index when compared to a usual diet group after three months (52).

The dietary supplement, Chlorella Pyrenoidosa, a phytonutrient derived from freshwater blue-green alga, has been tested in two clinical trials. An initial single group pilot study found a statistically significant decrease in pain intensity after 60 days of treatment. The follow-up RCT for three months found significant increases in global well being, sleep, and fatigue, and a trend toward pain relief in 43 FMS patients (53). Super Malic, a tablet containing malic acid [200 mg], an organic dicarboxylic acid, and magnesium [50 mg], was tested in a well-designed RCT study (54). No significant improvements in pain ratings during the blinded low-dose arm of the trial were reported, but significant improvements in pain and tenderness occurred during the dose-escalation open-label arm.

Two RCTs have explored the efficacy of S-adenosyl-L-methionine [SAMe] on symptoms of pain and depression in persons with FMS. In the first study (55), 44 subjects with FMS received a daily dose of oral SAMe 800 mg versus placebo for six weeks. Significant improvements were observed for pain, fatigue, and morning stiffness. In the second study (56), 34 subjects received a daily intravenous dose of SAMe 600 mg for 10 days with no significant effects. In the only RCT of guaifenesin (57), no significant effects on pain ratings, any other symptom, or laboratory measure was noted. The evidence for diet and supplement efficacy in FMS is mixed.

Magnets

Two RCTs using magnetic mattress pads for treatment of FMS have been completed. Significant pain relief, sleep improvement, and a decrease in FMS impact were found in the experimental group when compared to sham mattress control in one study (58). The second RCT concluded that, with the exception of pain intensity, the improvements in the experimental groups did not differ from the sham or usual care control groups (59). Thus, the evidence for the use of magnets in FMS treatment is inconsistent at this point.

EVALUATION AND RECOMMENDATIONS

Overall, there is moderate to strong evidence for the effectiveness of well-researched and accepted nonpharmacologic approaches to FMS treatment. Novel treatments from a wide group of practitioners and health perspectives are beginning to emerge as legitimate strategies.

Based on the current evidence, physical exercise that increases functional ability and education that includes both information and cognitive-behavioral strategies should be implemented in multicomponent programs. Since one of the most common significant outcomes is a change in self-efficacy, one of the goals of treatment should be to shift the patient's perception from one of helplessness and frustration to a positive sense of ability to perform desired behaviors.

A distinct limitation of the evidence base is the lack of trials that manipulate medications along with the nonpharmacologic treatments. Many trials make the point that drugs were monitored and attempts made to hold drug therapy constant during the clinical trial. However, an optimal individualized, treatment approach cannot be established without including medication management. More high quality RCTs with a drug component are necessary.

It is highly likely that both the well-researched approaches and novel approaches could be made more effective if subgroups of patients were identified and targeted with specific strategies early in the treatment process. Recent work has identified subgroups of FMS patients on the basis of psychosocial and behavioral responses to pain (60), fear of pain (61), and readiness to adopt a self-management approach to chronic pain (62). A diagnosis of FMS alone often results in heterogeneous research samples that generate weak or mixed outcomes to experimental treatment approaches.

A number of RCTs noted characteristics of subjects, who adhered to and completed the experimental treatment, responded to the experimental treatment, or maintained treatment gains at follow-up. Although adherence was measured in various ways, subjects who failed to complete the experimental treatments were more likely to have had a traumatic onset of FMS, missed work because of FMS symptoms, and scored lower at pretest on measures of perceived control over pain. Experimental treatment responders were more likely to be less depressed at pretest, have had pain for a shorter period of time, been physically active before entering the clinical trial, have a high sense of control over symptoms, an idiopathic onset of FMS symptoms, and social support from significant others. Maintenance of treatment gains was most clearly linked to continued performance of the skill learned in the experimental program [e.g., regular exercise] or continuing to access a treatment such as massage or balneotherapy. Research that identifies characteristics of patients who make long-term behavior changes and strategies to increase the likelihood that patients will make permanent changes in behaviors are needed.

REFERENCES

1. Busch A, Schachter CL, Peloso PM, Bombardier C: Exercise for treating fibromyalgia syndrome. Cochrane Database of Systematic Reviews 2004(1).

2. Mannerkorpi K, Iversen MD: Physical exercise in fibromyalgia and related syndromes. Best Practice Res Clin Rheumatol 17:629-647, 2003.

3. Williams DA: Psychological and behavioural therapies in fibromyalgia and related symptoms. Best Practice Res Clin Rheumatol 17:649-665, 2003.

4. Burckhardt CS, Bjelle A: Education programmes for fibromyalgia patients: Description and evaluation. Bailliere's Clin Rheumatol 8:935-956, 1994.

5. Karjalainen K, Malmivaara A, van Tulder M, Roine R, Jauhiainen M, Hurri H, Koes B: Multidisciplinary rehabilitation for fibromyalgia and musculoskeletal pain in working age adults. Cochrane Database of Systematic Reviews 2000(3).

6. Oliver K, Cronan TA, Walen HR: A review of multidisciplinary interventions for fibromyalgia patients: Where do we go from here? J Musculoskel Pain 9(4): 63-80, 2001.

7. Offenbaecher M, Stucki G: Physical therapy in the treatment of fibromyalgia. Scand J Rheumatol 29 (suppl 113):78-85, 2000.

8. Burckhardt CS: Nonpharmacologic management strategies in fibromyalgia. Rheum Dis Clin N Am 28: 291-304, 2002.

9. Rossy LA, Buckelew SP, Dorr N, Hagglund KJ, Thayer JF, McIntosh MJ, Hewett JE, Johnson JC: A meta-analysis of fibromyalgia treatment interventions. Ann Behav Med 21:180-191, 1999.

10. Sim J, Adams N: Systematic review of randomized controlled trails of nonpharmacological interventions for fibromyalgia. Clin J Pain 18:325-336, 2002.

11. Burckhardt CS, Mannerkorpi K, Hedenberg L, Bjelle A: A randomized, controlled clinical trial of education and physical training for women with fibromyalgia. J Rheumatol 21:714-720, 1994.

12. King S, Wessel J, Bhambhani Y, Sholter D, Maksymowch W: The effects of exercise and education, individually or combined, in women with fibromyalgia. J Rheumatol 29:2620-2627, 2002.

13. Oliver K, Cronan TA, Walen HR, Tomita M: Effects of social support and education on health care costs for patients with fibromyalgia. J Rheumatol 28:2711-2719, 2001.

14. Soares JF, Grossi G: A randomized controlled comparison of educational and behavioral interventions for women with fibromyalgia. Scand J Occup Ther 9:35-45, 2002.

15. Wigers SH, Stiles TC, Vogel PA: Effects of aerobic exercise versus stress management treatment in fibromyalgia. Scand J Rheumatol 25:77-86, 1996.

16. Vlaeyen JW, Teeken-Gruben NJ, Goossens ME, Rutten-vanMolken MPMH, Pelt RAGB, van Eek H, Heuts RHTG: Cognitive-educational treatment of fibromyalgia: a randomized clinical trial. I. Clinical effects. J Rheumatol 23:1237-1245, 1996.

17. Williams DA, Cary MA, Groner KH, Chaplin W, Glazer LJ, Rodriguez AM, Clauw DJ: Improving physical functional status in patients with fibromyalgia: A brief cognitive behavioral intervention. J Rheumatol 29:1280-1286, 2002.

18. Nicassio PM, Radojevic V, Weisman MH, Schuman C, Kim J, Schoenfeld-Smith K, Krall T: A comparison of behavioral and educational interventions for fibromyalgia. J Rheumatol 24:2000-2007, 1997.

19. Jones KD, Burckhardt CS, Clark SR, Bennett RM, Potempa K: A randomized controlled trial of muscle strengthening versus flexibility training in fibromyalgia. J Rheumatol 29:1041-1048, 2002.

20. Häkkinen A, Häkkinen K, Hannonen P, Alen M: Neuromuscular function of premenopausal women with fibromyalgia: Comparison with healthy women. Ann Rheum Dis 60:21-26, 2001.

21. Mannerkorpi K, Ahlmén M, Ekdahl C: Pool exercises combined with an education program for patients with fibromyalgia syndrome. A prospective, randomized study. J Rheumatol 27:2473-2481, 2000.

22. Richards SCM, Scott DL: Prescribed exercise in people with fibromyalgia: Parallel group randomised controlled trial. BMJ 325:185-187, 2002.

23. Cedraschi C, Desmeules J, Rapiti E, Baumgartner E, Cohen P, Finckh A, Allaz AF, Vischer TL: Fibromyalgia: A randomised, controlled trial of a treatment pro-

gramme based on self management. Ann Rheum Dis 63:290-296, 2004.

24. Buckelew SP, Conway R, Parker J: Biofeedback/relaxation training and exercise interventions for fibromyalgia: A prospective trial. Arthritis Care Res 11: 196-209, 1998.

25. Gowans SE, deHueck A, Voss S, Richardson M: A randomized, controlled trial of exercise and education for individuals with fibromyalgia. Arthritis Care Res 12:120-128, 1999.

26. Keel PJ, Bodoky C, Gerhard U, Muller W: Comparison of integrated group therapy and group relaxation training for fibromyalgia. Clin J Pain 14:232-238, 1998.

27. Bennett RM, Burckhardt CS, Clark SR, O'Reilly CA, Wiens AN, Campbell SM: Group treatment of fibromyalgia: a 6 month outpatient program. J Rheumatol 23:521-528, 1996.

28. Mengshoel AM, Haugen M: Health status in fibromyalgia–A followup study. J Rheumatol 28: 2085-2089, 2001.

29. Turk DC, Okifuji A, Sinclair JD, Starz TW: Interdisciplinary treatment for fibromyalgia syndrome: clinical and statistical significance. Arthritis Care Res 11:186-195, 1998.

30. White KP, Nielson WR: Cognitive behavioral treatment of fibromyalgia syndrome: A followup assessment. J Rheumatol 22:717-721, 1995.

31. Berman BM: Swyers JP: Complementary medicine treatments for fibromyalgia syndrome. Bailliere's Clin Rheumatol 13:487-492, 1999.

32. Crofford LJ, Appleton BE: Complementary and alternative therapies for fibromyalgia. Curr Rheumatol Rep 3:147-156, 2001.

33. Holdcraft LC, Assefin N, Buchwald D: Complementary and alternative medicine in fibromyalgia and related syndromes. Best Practice Res Clin Rheumatol 17:667-683, 2003.

34. Berman BM. Is acupuncture effective in the treatment of fibromyalgia? J Fam Pract 48:213-218, 1999.

35. DeLuze C, Bosia L, Zirb A, Chantraine A, Vischer TL: Electroacupuncture in fibromyalgia: Results of a controlled trial. BMJ 305:1249-1252, 1992.

36. Ferraccioli G, Ghirelli L, Scita F, Nolli M, Mozzani M, Fontana S, Scorsonelli M, Tridenti A, DeRisio C: EMG-biofeedback training in fibromyalgia syndrome. J Rheumatol 14:820-825, 1987.

37. Drexler AR, Mur EJ, Gunther VC: Efficacy of an EMG-biofeedback therapy in fibromyalgia patients. A comparative study of patients with and without abnormality in (MMPI) psychological scales. Clin Exp Rheumatol 20:677-682, 2002.

38. van Santen M, Bolwijn P, Verstappen F, Bakker C, Hidding A, Houben H, van der Heijde D, Landewe R, van der Linden S: A randomized clinical trial comparing fitness and biofeedback training versus basic treatment in patients with fibromyalgia. J Rheumatol 29:575-581, 2002.

39. Buskila D, Abu-Shakra M, Neumann L, Odes L, Shneider E, Flusser D, Sukenik, S: Balneotherapy for fibromyalgia at the Dead Sea. Rheumatol Int 20: 105-108, 2001.

40. Evcik D, Kizilay B, Gokcen E: The effects of balneotherapy on fibromyalgia patients. Rheumatol Int 22:56-59, 2002.

41. Ammer K, Melnizky P: Medicinal baths for treatment of generalized fibromyalgia. Forsch komplementarmed 6:80-85, 1999.

42. Altan L, Bingol U, Aykac M, Koc Z, Yurtkuran M: Investigation of the effects of pool-based exercise on fibromyalgia syndrome. Rheumatol Int 24 Sept, 2003.

43. Brattberg G: Connective tissue massage in the treatment of fibromyalgia. European J Pain 3:235-245, 1999.

44. Aslan UB, Yuksel I, Yazici M: A comparison of classical massage and mobilization techniques treatment in primary fibromyalgia. Fizyoterapi Rehabilitasyon 12(2):50-54, 2001.

45. Alnigenis MNY, Bradley JD, Wallick J, Emsley CL: Massage therapy in the management of fibromyalgia: A pilot study. J Musculoskel Pain 9(2):55-67, 2001.

46. Astin JA, Berman BM, Bausell B, Lee W-L, Hochberg MC, Forys KL: The efficacy of mindfulness meditation plus Qigong movement therapy in the treatment of fibromyalgia: A randomized controlled trial. J Rheumatol 30:2257-2262, 2003.

47. Kendall SA, Brolin-Magnusson K, Sörén B, Gerdle B, Henriksson KG: A pilot study of body awareness programs in the treatment of fibromyalgia syndrome. Arthritis Care Res 13:304-311, 2000.

48. Kendall SA, Ekselius L, Gerdle B, Sörén B, Bengtsson A: Feldenkrais intervention in fibromyalgia patients: A pilot study. J Musculoskel Pain 9(4):25-35, 2001.

49. Taggart HM, Arslanian CL, Bae S, Singh K: Effects of T'ai Chi exercise on fibromyalgia symptoms and health-related quality of life. Orthop Nurs 22: 353-560, 2003.

50. Creamer P, Singh BB, Hochberg MC, Berman BM: Sustained improvement produced by nonpharmacologic intervention in fibromyalgia: Results of a pilot study. Arthritis Care Res 13:198-204, 2000.

51. Azad KA, Alam MN, Haq SA, Nahar S, Chowdhury MA, Ali SM, Ullah AK: Vegetarian diet in the treatment of fibromyalgia. Bangladesh Med Res Counc Bull 26(2):41-47, 2000.

52. Kaartinen K, Lammi K, Hypen M, Nenonen M, Hänninen O, Rauma A-L: Vegan diet alleviates fibromyalgia symptoms. Scand J Rheumatol 29:308-313, 2000.

53. Merchant RE, Andre CA, Wise CM: Nutritional supplementation with Chlorella pyrenoidosa: A double-blind, placebo-controlled crossover study. J Musculoskel Pain 9(4):37-54, 2001.

54. Russell IJ, Michalek JE, Flechas JD, Abraham GE: Treatment of fibromyalgia syndrome with Super Malic: A randomized, double-blind, placebo controlled, crossover pilot study. J Rheumatol 22:953-958, 1995.

55. Jacobsen S, Danneskiold-Samsoe B, Andersen RB: Oral S-adenoslmethionine in primary fibromyalgia. Double-blind clinical evaluation. Scand J Rheumatol 20:294-302, 1991.

56. Volkman H, Norregaard J, Jacobsen S, Danneskiold-Samsoe B, Knoke G, Nehrdich D: Double-blind, placebo-controlled cross-over study of intravenous S-adenosyl-L-methionine in patients with fibromyalgia. Scand J Rheumatol 26:206-211, 1997.

57. Bennett RM, Clark SR: A randomized, prospective, 12 month study to compare the efficacy of guaifenesin versus placebo in the management of FMS. 2003, www.myalgia.com, accessed 10/22/03.

58. Colbert AP, Markov MS, Banerji M, Pilla AA: Magnetic mattress pad use in patients with fibromyalgia: A randomized double-blind pilot study. J Back Musculoskel Rehabil 13:19-31, 1999.

59. Alfano AP, Taylor AG, Foresman PA, Dunkl PR, McConnell GG, Conaway MR, Gillies GT: Static magnetic fields for treatment of fibromyalgia: A randomized controlled trial. J Altern Complement Med 7:53-64, 2001.

60. Turk DC, Okifuji A, Sinclair JD, Starz TW: Differential responses by psychosocial subgroups of fibromyalgia syndrome patients to an interdisciplinary treatment. Arthritis Care Res 11:297-404, 1998.

61. de Gier M, Peters ML, Vlaeyen JW: Fear of pain, physical performance and attentional processes in patients with fibromyalgia. Pain 104:121-130, 2003.

62. Jensen MP, Nielson WR, Turner JA, Romano JM, Hill ML: Readiness to self-manage pain is associated with coping and with psychological and physical functioning among patients with chronic pain. Pain 104: 529-537, 2003.

Fibromyalgia:
Novel Drug Therapies

Leslie Crofford

Objectives: Currently available pharmacologic agents used in the treatment of fibromyalgia syndrome [FMS] are often ineffective or poorly tolerated.

Methods: Several large randomized, placebo-controlled clinical trials of novel pharmacologic agents have been recently conducted in patients with FMS. Results of clinical trials using pregabalin, milnacipran, and duloxetine will be reviewed. The mechanism of action of these agents will be discussed. The design of each study and the study results will be reviewed.

Results: Treatment with pregabalin at the highest dose studies results in significant improvement in endpoint mean pain score as recorded in a daily diary. Pregabalin treatment was also associated with improvements in sleep, fatigue, patient and clinician global, and health related quality of life. Milnacipran administered in twice daily dose significantly lowered pain scores on binary and continuous pain score analyses. Milnacipran-treated patients also improved in multiple components of the fibromyalgia impact questionnaire [FIQ] and on patient global assessment. Duloxetine was studied in FMS patients with and without depression. Significant improvement in the FIQ total, but not the FIQ pain score, were seen in the duloxetine-treated group. Other pain measures were significantly improved. Improvements were seen regardless of depression status at baseline and treatment effects were significantly greater in female patients.

Conclusions: Novel drugs are in development for use in the FMS population and have been found efficacious for pain and other symptoms of FMS. It will be important to develop outcome measures for use in clinical trials. It is expected that the development of new drugs will bring more effective treatment that will be applied earlier in the course of disease. This may bring us closer to the goal of improving health-related quality of life for patients with FMS.

Leslie Crofford, MD, was with the University of Michigan, Ann Arbor, MI. Currently she is affiliated with the University of Kentucky, Lexington, KY.

[Haworth co-indexing entry note]: "Fibromyalgia: Novel Drug Therapies." Crofford, Leslie. Co-published simultaneously in *Journal of Musculoskeletal Pain* [The Haworth Medical Press, an imprint of The Haworth Press, Inc.] Vol. 12, No. 3/4, 2004, p. 73; and: *Soft Tissue Pain Syndromes: Clinical Diagnosis and Pathogenesis* [ed: Dieter E. Pongratz, Siegfried Mense, and Michael Spaeth] The Haworth Medical Press, an imprint of The Haworth Press, Inc., 2004, p. 73. Single or multiple copies of this article are available for a fee from The Haworth Document Delivery Service [1-800-HAWORTH, 9:00 a.m. - 5:00 p.m. [EST]. E-mail address: docdelivery@haworthpress.com].

Available online at http://www.haworthpress.com/web/JMP
doi:10.1300/J094v12n03_11

Painful Myopathies–
Metabolism of Muscle Cells and Metabolic Myopathies

Heinz Reichmann
Jochen Schaefer

SUMMARY. Myalgias may be caused by intrinsic muscular factors [inflammation, mechanical disturbances, ischemia, metabolic abnormalities, membrane alterations] or by extrinsic factors like diseases of the peripheral or central nervous system. Primary metabolic myopathies are mostly caused by disturbances of energy metabolism. Usually these patients present with exercise-induced myalgia, which is commonly associated with muscle weakness. If rhabdomyolysis occurs further thorough investigations for a metabolic myopathy are mandatory. The pathogenesis of myalgia is thought to be related to certain biochemical mediators. Disturbances of anaerobic and aerobic muscle metabolism are typical for metabolic myopathies causing myalgia. These disorders are due to enzyme malfunction in the following pathways: glycogenolysis, glycolysis, β-oxidation of fatty acids, and the respiratory chain. Treatment of metabolic myopathies is limited. Non-specific measures include physiotherapy, non-steroidal analgesics, chinine, and L-carnitine. It is essential, however, to avoid endurance exercise with abnormalities of aerobic metabolism and to avoid brief intensive exercise with disturbances of anaerobic metabolism. *[Article copies available for a fee from The Haworth Document Delivery Service: 1-800-HAWORTH. E-mail address: <docdelivery@ haworthpress.com> Website: <http://www.HaworthPress.com> © 2004 by The Haworth Press, Inc. All rights reserved.]*

KEYWORDS. Myalgia, etiology, metabolic myopathy, metabolism

CLASSIFICATION OF MYALGIAS

Myalgias are one of the most prominent features of neuromuscular diseases. It is thought that up to three percent of the population may suffer from myalgia (1). It may be caused by disturbances of muscle [primary myalgia], neurons and nerve roots [secondary myalgia]. In addi-

Heinz Reichmann, Prof. Dr. med., and Jochen Schaefer, MD, are affiliated with the Department of Neurology, University of Dresden, Fetscherstraße 74, D-01307 Dresden, Germany [E-mail: schaefer@rcs.urz.tu-dresden.de].

[Haworth co-indexing entry note]: "Painful Myopathies–Metabolism of Muscle Cells and Metabolic Myopathies." Reichmann, Heinz, and Jochen Schaefer. Co-published simultaneously in *Journal of Musculoskeletal Pain* [The Haworth Medical Press, an imprint of The Haworth Press, Inc.] Vol. 12, No. 3/4, 2004, pp. 75-83; and: *Soft Tissue Pain Syndromes: Clinical Diagnosis and Pathogenesis* [ed: Dieter E. Pongratz, Siegfried Mense, and Michael Spaeth] The Haworth Medical Press, an imprint of The Haworth Press, Inc., 2004, pp. 75-83. Single or multiple copies of this article are available for a fee from The Haworth Document Delivery Service [1-800-HAWORTH, 9:00 a.m. - 5:00 p.m. [EST]. E-mail address: docdelivery@haworthpress.com].

tion, even central nervous system disease may cause secondary myalgia due to spasticity, rigidity, dystonia, or tetanus. It is helpful to subdivide myalgia into focal and diffuse types and paroxysmal myalgia [Table 1]. Paroxysmal myalgia is typically associated with cramps and spasms.

Careful analysis of aggravating and relieving factors is helpful for establishing the diagnosis. Metabolic myopathies are characterized by their association with exercise [exertional muscle pain syndrome]; the myalgias are commonly reported as stiffness thereby causing hampered limb movements.

Myalgias may be caused by mechanical damage such as excentric muscle contraction [e.g., down-hill walking, jumping from a chair] (2,3), haematoma and compartment syndromes; further by inflammatory lesions, ischaemic muscle infarcts, metabolic myopathies, and other myopathies like dystrophies and myotonias.

It is sometimes difficult to differentiate myalgias from joint pains. A typical example is quadriceps muscle pain due to coxarthrosis. Passive joint movements will be painful in case of an underlying arthropathy, but they will not exacerbate myogenic pain.

TABLE 1

Characteristics of Myalgia	Cause of Myalgia
Focal muscle pain	Haematoma, pyomyositis, Infarction of muscle, alcohol myopathy, compartment syndromes, restless-legs syndrome, neurogenic pain
Diffuse muscle pain	Polymyositis, necrotising myopathy [alcohol, drugs, electrolyte disturbances], fibromyalgia, polymyalgia rheumatica
Paroxysmal muscle pain	
Cramps in healthy individuals	Overload, cramp in calf muscles at night, electrolyte disturbances, dehydration
Cramps in neuromuscular diseases	Neurogenic causes [amyotrophic lateral sclerosis, polyneuropathies, radiculopathies], systemic disturbances due to renal or liver diseases, hypothyroidism, hyperthyroidism
Contractures	Enzyme defects in glycogenolysis, glycolysis, Brody's disease, rippling-muscle disease, hypothyroidism
Myotonia	Channelopathies, proximal myotonic myopathy
Exercise-induced muscle pain	Glycogenoses, defects of glycolysis, defects of lipid metabolism, mitochondrial myopathies, myoadenylate deaminase deficiency, dystrophinopathies

ENERGY METABOLISM IN MUSCLE

Since disturbances of muscular energy metabolism represent one of the most important causes of myalgia, the physiology of muscle metabolism will be described here.

Adenosine-triphosphate [ATP] is the "fuel" for muscle function, and this is the reason why energy metabolism is geared towards the production of ATP. Two main pathways are involved in ATP production, the aerobic and anaerobic degradation of glycogen and glucose and the aerobic degradation of lipids [Figure 1].

Glycolysis is located in the cytoplasm and performs the function of anaerobic glucose energy metabolism, whilst the citric acid cycle and respiratory chain are located in the mitochondria and perform aerobic glucose energy metabolism [oxidative phosphorylation]. Anaerobic glycolytic degradation of one mole of glucose yields two moles of ATP, whilst aerobic degradation of one mole of glucose yields 36 moles of ATP. The degradation of one mole of palmitic acid yields 131 moles of ATP.

In addition to these pathways, adenosine-diphosphate [ADP] can be directly converted to ATP by transferring a phosphate group from creatine phosphate. This reaction is catalysed by creatine kinase. On the whole, this pathway does not supply the muscle with much ATP, but guarantees a constant ATP level within the first minute of muscle action. Thereafter, glucose and fatty acids are required for energy supply.

At rest, during prolonged fasting or during moderate exercise the energy demands are mostly met by fatty acid degradation. During fast and highly strenuous exercise glycogen and glucose are the most important energy suppliers. During continuous low-intensity exercise fatty acid degradation [beta-oxidation of fatty acids] is essential and supplies the muscle with more than 60 percent of its energy requirements. Depending on the energy demand the reaction velocities of these pathways may increase up to 100 fold (4).

Due to their higher energy yield fatty acids are more important than carbohydrates as metabolic fuels. The amount of fatty acids stored in fat depots by far exceeds the amount of all the body's stores of carbohydrates. Fatty acid beta-oxidation is located in the mitochondria and is part of aerobic metabolism, which implies that

FIGURE 1. Mitochondrial energy metabolism

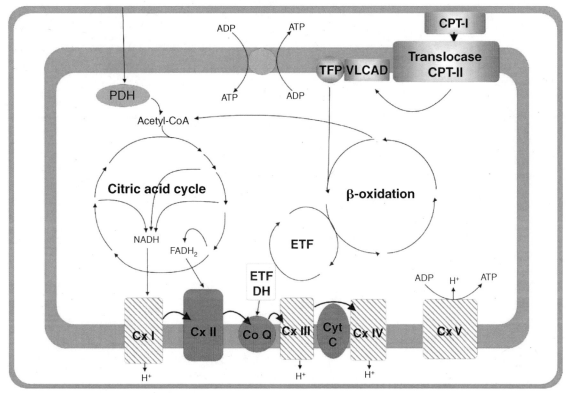

PDH: Pyruvate dehydrogenase)
CPT: Carnitine palmitoyltransferase) fatty acid β-
VLCAD: Very long-chain acyl-CoA-dehydrogenase) oxidation
TFP: Trifunctional protein of β-oxidation)
ETF: Electron transfer flavoprotein)

Cx I-V: Complex I-V)
CoQ: Coenzyme Q10) respiratory
Cyt C: Cytochrome C) chain

oxygen is required for the degradation of free fatty acids. Since the fatty acid stores of muscle fibers are limited, they have to be released from the fat depots of the body by lipolysis. They are transported to the muscle through the bloodstream bound to albumin. Free fatty acids require a special carnitine-dependent transporter system [carnitine palmityltransferase, carnitine translocase] to permeate the mitochondrial membranes before they undergo a cyclic degradation process called beta-oxidation of fatty acids [Figure 1]. The end product, acetyl-CoA, is identical to the one created by glucose degradation. Acetyl-CoA is further oxidised to CO_2 and water in the citric acid cycle. The redox potential created by these pathways is transferred to the respiratory chain via NADH and $FADH_2$. The respiratory chain is the final common pathway and consists of five complexes which are incorporated into the mitochondrial inner membrane. The respiratory chain is the site of ATP synthesis.

Glucose may also be degraded by glycolysis which is 18 times less efficient than degradation by aerobic metabolism. Anaerobic degradation of glucose yields pyruvate which is further reduced to lactate in order to regenerate NAD. Lactate levels increase during exercise and are a parameter of the anaerobic metabolism of glycogen and glucose. In the aerobic pathway pyruvate is metabolised to acetyl-CoA by pyruvate dehydrogenase which is then fed into the citric acid cycle and the respiratory chain [Figure 1].

Glucose is stored in muscle as glycogen and is therefore available at the site of action in muscle fibers. Glycogenolysis is initiated by a reaction catalysed by myo-phosphorylase which releases glucose-1-phosphate from the glycogen molecule. All enzymes of glycolysis are present in the cytoplasm and permit degradation of glucose-1-phosphate by the glycolytic pathway after conversion to glucose-6-phosphate. Muscular glycogen stores are sufficient for three minutes of maximal muscular exercise (6), whilst the capacity of triglycerides is almost unlimited.

These biochemical features are not only the basis for understanding myalgia in metabolic myopathies, but also indicate ways to avoid exercise-induced myalgia.

PATHOGENESIS OF MUSCLE PAIN IN METABOLIC MYOPATHIES

The sensory functions of muscle are still not completely understood. It is thought that myalgia does not develop in the muscle parenchyma but in the endo- and perimysial structures as well as in the fascias and tendon insertions. Nociceptors located in these structures conduct pain via unmyelinated C-fibers and thinly myelinated $A\delta$-fibers to the central nervous system. Nociceptors are stimulated by mechanical or chemical stimuli. They may be unimodal or polymodal, i.e., they can either be stimulated by only one specific stimulus or by many. Basically, chemical stimuli give rise to slowly progressive continuous dull pain, whilst mechanical stimuli cause short-lasting sharp pain sensations (7). The most aggressive chemical stimuli known

so far are bradykinine, serotonine, histamine, adenosine, inosine-monophosphate, phosphate, potassium ions, and H_3O^+ ions. Adenosine is released in high amounts in ischaemic muscle and is considered to be one of the most important pain inductors. Myalgia due to ischaemia can be significantly reduced by caffeine, an adenosine antagonist (8), whereas intra-arterial injection of adenosine causes typical muscle pain (9).

Lactate is probably not a sufficient stimulus for pain in metabolic myopathies. This is underlined by the fact that the extremely painful contractures of McArdle syndrome are not associated with increased lactate levels.

In contrast, the significance of tissue pH for myalgia is undisputed and was confirmed in some experiments: intramuscular infusion of acidic phosphate buffer [pH 5.2] leads to a linear increase of pain, comparable to the pain observed in muscle ischaemia (10). In contrast, there is no decrease in muscle pH in McArdle disease despite intense pain (7).

Corresponding to the polymodality of most nociceptors it is reasonable to assume that the biochemically diverse metabolic myopathies utilize different mediators to transmit pain. So far, no such mediator could be found in any metabolic myopathy.

There are, however, other possibilities for the development of pain: it may be that specific intermediates of energy metabolism could cause pain by increasing the sensitivity of nociceptors. Thus, they may over-respond to otherwise normal mechanical stimuli such as muscular exercise. This may be one of the causes of pain in fibromyalgia (11) and also in metabolic myopathies. The similar character of the pain in metabolic myopathies and in muscle overuse [muscle soreness] corroborates this assumption. Muscle soreness is most probably caused by mechanical microruptures of the sarcomeric structures followed by metabolic reactions (12). This explains the frequently observed delay in the occurrence of pain in metabolic myopathies [delay until the secondary reactions have started or finished]. As in other pain syndromes central factors [neuroplasticity, pain memory] and psychosocial factors also play a role in muscle pain. These additional factors are thought to be causal for chronic pain [Figure 2].

FIGURE 2. Metabolic myopathies

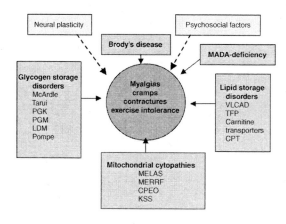

MUSCLE PAIN IN METABOLIC MYOPATHIES

Typically, metabolic myopathies are associated with diffuse exercise-induced myalgia and contractures [Table 1]. Usually pain is also associated with short-lasting muscle weakness. Focal or diffuse muscle pain without corresponding muscle weakness points against a metabolic myopathy, and in many cases a clear-cut diagnosis is impossible. In a retrospective study of 100 patients with diffuse and exercise-induced muscular pain. a muscle biopsy allowed a distinct diagnosis in only five patients (13): two patients suffered from polymyositis with elevated creatine kinase [CK] levels, two from McArdle syndrome [with elevated CK and a myopathic pattern in the electromyogram [EMG]], and one from a mitochondrial myopathy. Approximately 25 percent of the patients showed non-specific findings such as myopathic changes, type II fiber disproportion and single fiber necroses which did not allow a diagnosis. In contrast, if muscle weakness and particularly elevations of CK and rhabdomyolysis co-occur a myopathy can frequently be diagnosed (14). If muscle weakness and rhabdomyolysis are strictly related to exercise a metabolic myopathy is the most likely diagnosis. These observations are in agreement with the clinical experience that diffuse muscle pain, even if it is exacerbated by exercise, can only be attributed to a diagnosis if there are additional symptoms, neurophysiological or biochemical findings.

Cramps

Many patients with metabolic myopathies complain of muscle cramps, although true cramps are caused by neurogenic and not by myopathic disease. Muscle cramps can present with painful visible or palpable focal muscle contractions frequently leading to abnormal joint positions which are improved by passive stretching of the muscle. In an EMG the contracted muscle shows high-frequency discharges and normal action potentials. Cramps are induced by ephaptic discharges of central or peripheral segments of the motorneurons. Common causes of cramps are polyneuropathy, radiculopathy, motor neurone disease and disturbances of electrolytes [particularly magnesium and calcium] and water balance. Cramps also occur in healthy individuals both at rest and after strenuous exercise. In any case, cramps are a neurogenic phenomenon.

Contractures

The character of the pain is very similar in contractures and cramps. Contractures, however, never occur at rest, but only after repetitive muscle contractions. The main difference is that contractures are silent in the EMG whilst cramps are not. The most relevant disorders leading to contractures are defects of glycolysis such as McArdle's syndrome and deficiency of phosphofructokinase [PFK]. Other impairments of energy metabolism like beta-oxidation defects or defects of the respiratory chain never cause contractures. Thus, it can be speculated that the lack of lactate increase which is typical of glycolytic defects, may be the cause for contractures. Ruff et al. (15) performed experiments in which the inhibition of glycolysis and creatine kinase resulted in a massive rise of ADP, which increased the binding of myosin to actin filaments thereby inducing contractures. Other disturbances of muscle relaxation may also cause contractures [Table 1]. Examples are Brody's disease, hypothyroidism, and ripplingmuscle disease.

Myotonia

Myotonia is characterised by prolonged muscle contraction and delayed relaxation and is caused by altered properties of the sarcolemma.

Myotonia is not seen in metabolic myopathies, but is typical of hereditary channelopathies, proximal myotonic myopathy, or myotonic dystrophy. These patients mostly complain of muscle stiffness and sometimes of painful muscle cramps.

Exercise-Induced Myalgia

If patients complain of exercise-induced myalgia metabolic myopathies should be suspected first. The onset of myalgia during muscular activity may help to differentiate between the underlying defects: muscle contractions with high force and frequency require glycolysis–therefore, such an enzyme defect will cause muscle pain in combination with muscle weakness and contractures if such demands are made. Conversely, exercise-related myalgia may occur in mitochondrial enzyme defects if prolonged strenuous exercise is performed. Unfortunately, even extended diagnostic procedures sometimes fail to lead to a definite diagnosis in patients with exercise-induced myalgia. Such patients very often have slightly elevated CK activities, myopathic patterns in the EMG, and non-specific changes in a muscle biopsy like tubular aggregates (16) or a reduced number of type I fibers (17).

SPECIFIC DISEASES

A detailed discussion of all muscle disorders can be found in text books and reviews (e.g., 5,18-20).

Defects of Glycogenolysis and Glycolysis

Acid Maltase Deficiency

A deficiency of acid maltase, a lysosomal enzyme which releases glucose from glycogen and maltose, causes proximal muscle weakness, joint contractures, and weakness of the respiratory muscles [Pompe's disease] in infancy. Patients who develop this myopathy during adolescence or in adulthood, also present with proximal muscle weakness and resemble patients with limb girdle muscular dystrophy. Exercise-induced myalgia may also occur in some of these patients. Muscle biopsy reveals a vacuolar myopathy with glycogen storage.

McArdle Syndrome

This disease is caused by a defect of muscle phosphorylase which cleaves glycosyl-moieities from glycogen. Patients can manage mild exercise like walking, but they cannot run fast or climb stairs without precipitating painful muscle contractures which make them abandon the exercise. Episodic exercise-induced muscle weakness and rhabdomyolysis occur frequently. Disease progression is usually slow, and only a third of the patients show fast deterioration. A typical finding is the so-called "second-wind phenomenon" which is characterized by the disappearance of the myalgias after temporary interruption and subsequent resumption of the exercise [switch to aerobic beta-oxidation]. The diagnosis is made by histochemistry, biochemistry, and by the ischaemic forearm test.

Defects in Phosphofructokinase [Tarui Disease]

Phosphofructokinase converts fructose-6-phosphate to fructose-1,6-diphosphate using ATP. Phosphofructokinase is a rate-limiting enzyme of glycolysis. The clinical picture resembles McArdle syndrome with exercise-induced contractures and myalgia. Ignoring the myalgia may lead to dangerous rhabdomyolysis with myoglobinuria and renal failure. Many patients carry the enzyme defect not only in their muscle but also in their red blood cells which leads to haemolytic anemia. Patients with PFK deficiency also demonstrate a second-wind phenomenon. Ingestion of glucose exacerbates the symptoms due to the accumulation of non-degradable intermediates. Diagnosis is based on the lack of histochemical staining for PFK and a pathological ischaemic lactate test.

Other enzyme defects such as aldolase, phosphoglycerate kinase, phosphoglycerate mutase, and lactate dehydrogenase are extremely rare and also present with exercise-induced contractures and rhabdomyolysis.

Defects of Lipid Metabolism

Beta-oxidation of free fatty acids is used for prolonged exercise and during fasting. In addition, fatty acid oxidation produces important metabolic intermediates like acetyl-CoA and reducing equivalents to maintain hepatic gluconeogenesis. The clinical presentations of the various defects of beta-oxidation resemble each other and therefore only permit prediction of the correct diagnosis in a few special cases. In children, defects of beta-oxidation lead to liver abnormalities, whereas they cause mostly muscle symptoms in adults. After prolonged exertion these patients develop severe myalgia, muscle weakness, stiffness, and contractures. Myoglobinuria may occur after a delay of several hours. Fasting, cold, and dehydration due to fever are additional risk factors for the development of rhabdomyolysis and renal failure. Cardiac involvement is possible. Analysis of fatty acid oxidation intermediates by mass spectrometry is mandatory. More frequently occuring deficiencies involve carnitine palmitoyltransferase, medium-chain acyl-CoA dehydrogenase, very long-chain acyl-CoA dehydrogenase, and the plasmalemmal carnitine transporter. An extensive discussion of these diseases can be found in (19).

Defects of the Respiratory Chain Enzymes

Although the respiratory chain is one of the most important aerobic pathways, patients with defects of one or more respiratory chain enzymes rarely complain of myalgia or exercise-induced muscle weakness. Due to the involvement of many organs the patients consider myalgia as one of their minor symptoms. Muscle function is impaired by excessive fatigue and to a lesser degree by myalgia. An exception to this rule are mutations in the gene for cytochrome b where myalgias and muscle weakness are the key symptoms. The lack of myalgia despite the presence of elevated lactate levels once again emphasises the theory that increased lactate concentrations do not cause myalgia per se.

Chronic Progressive External Ophthalmoplegia

These patients present with progressive external ophthalmoplegia with ptosis and only mild painless muscle weakness. Patients who are younger than 20 years and present with ataxia, pigmentary retinopathy and cardiac conduction defects suffer from Kearns-Sayre-syndrome. Both syndromes are caused by mutations or deletions of the mitochondrial genome.

Mitochondrial Myopathy, Encephalopathy, Lactate Acidosis and Stroke-Like Episodes [MELAS]

Like the myoclonic encephalopathy with ragged-red-fibers [MERRF] syndrome, the MELAS syndrome is predominantly characterized by symptoms due to the involvement of the central nervous system. Both diseases are caused by point mutations of the mitochondrial genome (5).

Brody's Disease

Brody's disease is a rare condition which is caused by a deficiency of sarcoplasmic Ca^{2+}-ATPase. This defect leads to an impairment of calcium re-uptake after muscle contraction which results in prolonged contraction and impaired relaxation. Repetitive muscle contraction can therefore cause contractures. Normally, these patients complain of exercise-induced myalgia and stiffness which looks myotonic. In contrast to typical myotonia, however, repetitive muscle activity does not induce muscle relaxation but even more severe contraction. Electromyogram analyses do not show myotonic discharges and CK levels are usually normal.

Deficiency of Myoadenylate Deaminase [MADA]

Myoadenylate deaminase catalyses the deamination of adenosine monophosphate to inosine monophosphate with release of ammonia. Clinically, deficiency of MADA manifests itself as exercise-induced myalgia and cramps (23). The disease is caused by nonsense mutations of the MADA gene. Since some homozygous mutation carriers are symptom-free, controversy surrounds this disease (24), and there are still some doubts whether it actually represents a separate disease entity.

THERAPY OF MYALGIAS CAUSED BY METABOLIC MYOPATHIES

Specific Therapy

The treatment of myalgias due to metabolic myopathies is based on the treatment of the underlying enzyme defect.

All patients with a defect of glucose metabolism should have a protein-rich diet (18). The benefit of glucose and fructose with regard to exercise tolerance in patients with McArdle's syndrome is controversial (25). Glucose supplementation is not helpful for patients with PFK deficiency. In general, mild exercise is recommended, taking into account the plasma CK values (26).

In contrast to defects of anaerobic energy metabolism, disturbances of beta-oxidation can be treated more effectively by:

- avoidance of fasting and prolonged exercise,
- carbohydrate-rich diet [70 percent] with low fat content [< 20 percent],
- medium-chain triglyceride supplements in patients with defects of long-chain fatty acid oxidation, and
- supplementation of L-carnitine and riboflavin in some patients (19).

As discussed for the glycolytic defects, there is also no causal therapy for defects of the respiratory chain. Most neurologists use a cocktail of vitamins and coenzyme Q10 in addition to a low-carbohydrate and high-lipid diet (5). Verapamil is effective in Brody's disease (27).

Non-Specific Therapy

Non-specific therapy includes physiotherapy and drug treatment. Using a diary allows the patient to assess which type of exercise is harmful. Depending on the affected metabolic pathway [aerobic or anaerobic] the most suitable sport disciplines have to be selected (26). Warming-up exercises, physical therapy, and dietary measures are helpful. L-carnitine was used with some success for myalgia due to excentric muscle contraction (28). The most important measure, however, is to tell the patient how to deal with their energy impairment and to avoid overuse of their muscles.

REFERENCES

1. Goldenberg GL: Fibromyalgia syndrome–An emerging but controversial condition. J Amer Med Ass 257: 2782-2787, 1987.

2. Newham DJ, McPhail G, Mills KR, Edwards RHT: Ultrastructural changes after concentric and excentric contractions of human muscle. J Neurol Sci 61: 109-122, 1983.

3. Gleeson M, Almey J, Brooks S, Cave R, Lewis A, Griffiths H: Hematological and acute-phase responses associated with delayed-onset muscle soreness in humans. Eur J Appl Physiol 71: 137-142, 1995.

4. Gibala MJ, MacLean DA, Graham TE, Saltin B: Tricarboxylic acid intermediate pool size and estimated cycle flux in human muscle during exercise. Am J Physiol 38: 235-242, 1998.

5. Schmiedel J, Jackson S, Schaefer J, Reichmann H: Mitochondrial cytopathies. J Neurol 250: 267-277, 2003.

6. Casey A, Short AH, Hultman E, Greenhaff PL: Glycogen resynthesis in human muscle fibre types following exercise-induced glycogen depletion. J Physiol 483: 265-271, 1995.

7. Mills KR, Newham DJ, Edwards RHT: Muscle pain. In: Textbook of pain (Wall PD, Melzak R, eds.). New York: Churchill-Livingstone, pp. 319-330, 1985.

8. Myers DE, Shaikh Z, Zullo TG: Hypoalgesic effect of caffeine in experimental ischemic muscle contraction pain. Headache 37: 654-658, 1997.

9. Sylven C, Jonzon B, Fedholm BB, Kaijser L: Adenosine injection into the brachial artery produces ischemia-like pain of discomfort in the forearm. Cardiovasc Res 22: 674-678, 1988.

10. Issberner U, Reeh PW, Steen KH: Pain due to tissue acidosis–A mechanism for inflammatory and ischaemic myalgia? Neurosci Lett 208: 191-194, 1996.

11. Soernson J, Graven-Nielsen T, Henriksson KG, Bengtsson M, Arendt-Nielsen L: Hyperexcitability in fibromyalgia. J Rheumatol 25: 152-155, 1998.

12. Friden J: Muscle soreness after exercise: Implications of morphological changes. Int J Sports Med 5: 57-66, 1984.

13. Pourmand R: The value of muscle biopsy in myalgia. Neurolgist 3: 173-177, 1997.

14. Mills KR, Edwards RHT: Investigative strategies for muscle pain. J Neurol Sci 58: 57-66, 1983.

15. Ruff RL, Weissman J: Possible role of ADP in contracture of muscle with impaired myoglycolysis. Neurology 39: 360, 1989.

16. Danon MJ, Carpenter S, Harati Y: Muscle pain associated with tubular aggregates and structures resembling cylindrical spirals. Muscle&Nerve 12: 265-272, 1989.

17. Lane RJM, Turnbull DM, Welch JL, Walton JN: A double-blind, placebo-controlled, crossover study of verapamil in exertional muscle pain syndrom. Muscle&Nerve 9: 635-641, 1986.

18. DiMauro S, Tsujino S: Non-lysosomal Glycogenoses. In: Myology. Engel AG, Franzini-Armstron C (eds.), McGraw-Hill, New York, pp. 1554-1576,1994.

19. Schaefer J, Pourfarzam, Bartlett K, Jackson S, Turnbull DM: Fatty acid oxidation in peripheral blood cells: Characterization and use for the diagnosis of defects of fatty acid oxidation. Pediatr Res 37: 354-360, 1995.

20. DiMauro S, Bonilla E: Mitochondrial encephalomyopathies. In: Rosenberg RN, Prusiner SB, DiMauro S, Barchi RL (eds.). The molecular and genetic basis of neurological diseases. Boston Wellington: Butterworth Heinemann, pp. 201-235, 1997.

21. Andreu AL, Hanna MG, Reichmann H, et al.: Exercise intolerance due to mutations in the cytochrome b gene of mitochondrial DANN. N Engl J Med 341: 1037-1044, 1999.

22. Betz RC, Schoser BG, Kasper D, et al.: Mutations in caveolin-r cause mechanical hyperirritability of skeletal muscle in rippling muscle disease. Nat Genet 28: 218-219, 2001.

23. Verzijl AT, van Engelen G, Luyten JA, et al.: Genetic characteristics of myoadenylate deaminase deficiency. Ann Neurol 44: 140-143, 1998.

24. Fishbein WN: Primary, secondary and coincidental types of myoadenylate deaminase deficiency. Ann Neurol 45: 547-548, 1999.

25. Tein I: Neonatal metabolic myopathies. Sem Perinatol 23: 125-151, 1999.

26. Schaefer J, Reichmann H. Sport bei metabolischen Myopathien. Akt Neurol 28: 26-30, 2001.

27. Taylor DJ, Brosnan MJ, Arnold DL, et al.: Ca^{2+}-ATPase deficiency in a patient with exertional muscle pain syndrome. J Neurol Neurosurg Psych 51: 1425-1433, 1988.

28. Giamberardino MA, Drtagani L, Valente R, et al.: Effects of prolonged L-carnitine administration on delayed muscle pain and CK release after excentric effort. Inter J Sports Med 17: 320-324, 1996.

29. Hultman E, Sjöholm H, Jaederholm EI, et al.: Evaluation of methods for electrical stimulation of human skeletal muscle in situ. Pflügers Arch 398: 139-141, 1983.

Clinical Presentation and Therapy
of Idiopathic Inflammatory Myopathies

Frederick W. Miller

SUMMARY. The idiopathic inflammatory myopathies [IIM] are a group of systemic immune-mediated disorders characterized by chronic muscle weakness and inflammation. The most common forms are polymyositis, dermatomyositis, and inclusion body myositis; however, dividing the IIM into serologic groups is also useful for assessing and managing these syndromes. Although pathogeneses are unknown, evidence suggests that these acquired diseases result from environmental exposures in genetically susceptible individuals.

Clinical presentations are quite diverse and range from slowly progressive nearly asymptomatic syndromes to acute life-threatening disorders. Signs and symptoms vary widely and often change over the course of the illness. Common signs and symptoms include: fatigue, muscle pain and atrophy, arthralgia and arthritis, rashes of many types, shortness of breath, dysphagia, edema, Raynaud's phenomenon, subcutaneous nodules and calcifications, dysphonia, fever, gastrointestinal pain, and weight loss.

Therapy has been poorly studied due to the rarity and heterogeneity of IIM. The goals of therapy are to eliminate inflammation in involved tissues and to regain function through rehabilitation. Corticosteroids remain first line therapy, although in cases with poor prognostic features, additional immunosuppressives are often used from the beginning of disease. Methotrexate, azathioprine, and intravenous immunoglobulin are the best-studied agents, but other drugs reported to be useful include cyclosporin, tacrolimus, cyclophosphamide, hydroxychloroquine sulfate, mycophenolate mofetil, and combinations of the above. Case reports suggest that targeted biologic agents, including monoclonal antibodies or fusion proteins directed at TNF alpha, B cells or complement, as well as autologous stem cell transplantation, might be beneficial and research is ongoing in this area. Advances in understanding the pathology and immunology of myositis, the development of new agents for related conditions, and recent international consensus on the conduct and reporting of myositis clinical trials, should all add momentum to improving outcomes for these increasingly recognized disorders. *[Article copies available for a fee from The Haworth Document Delivery Service: 1-800-HAWORTH. E-mail address: <docdelivery@haworthpress.com> Website: <http://www.HaworthPress.com>]*

KEYWORDS. Myositis, polymyositis, dermatomyositis, inclusion body myositis, therapy

INTRODUCTION

The idiopathic inflammatory myopathies [IIM] are a diverse collection of systemic connective tissue diseases currently defined by characteristic clinical, biochemical, histopathologic, electrophysiologic, and immunologic abnormalities (1). They are poorly studied in all

Frederick W. Miller, MD, PhD, is Chief, Environmental Autoimmunity Group, Office of Clinical Research, National Institute of Environmental Health Sciences, National Institutes of Health, 9000 Rockville Pike, NIH Building 9, Room 1W107, MSC 0958, Bethesda, MD 20892-0958 USA [E-mail: millerf@mail.nih.gov].

[Haworth co-indexing entry note]: "Clinical Presentation and Therapy of Idiopathic Inflammatory Myopathies." Miller, Frederick W. Co-published simultaneously in *Journal of Musculoskeletal Pain* [The Haworth Medical Press, an imprint of The Haworth Press, Inc.] Vol. 12, No. 3/4, 2004, pp. 85-91; and: *Soft Tissue Pain Syndromes: Clinical Diagnosis and Pathogenesis* [ed: Dieter E. Pongratz, Siegfried Mense, and Michael Spaeth] The Haworth Medical Press, an imprint of The Haworth Press, Inc., 2004, pp. 85-91. Single or multiple copies of this article are available for a fee from The Haworth Document Delivery Service [1-800-HAWORTH, 9:00 a.m. - 5:00 p.m. [EST]. E-mail address: docdelivery@haworthpress.com].

Available online at http://www.haworthpress.com/web/JMP
doi:10.1300/J094v12n03_13

aspects, but appear to be increasing in frequency over the last several decades. The pathogeneses of these illnesses, which consist of the major clinical groups of polymyositis [PM], dermatomyositis [DM] and inclusion body myositis [IBM], are unknown however, evidence suggests that these acquired diseases result from chronic immune activation following environmental exposures in genetically susceptible individuals (2,3).

In addition to the clinical groups above, these syndromes can also be classified by immune responses, which are either specific for myositis [the myositis-specific autoantibodies] or are associated with myositis [the myositis-associated autoantibodies]. The three major myositis-specific autoantibodies are autoantibodies directed against the aminoacyl-tRNA synthetases [anti-synthetases], proteins of the signal recognition particle [anti-SRP], and a nuclear helicase [anti-Mi-2] (4). Dividing these heterogeneous disorders into immune response groups results in more homogeneous subsets in terms of clinical presentation, genetics, epidemiology, responses to therapy, and prognosis (5).

Table 1 summarizes important features of the major IIM clinical and serologic groups.

CLINICAL PRESENTATION

The myositis syndromes present in a wide variety of ways. Myositis may develop acutely, subacutely or insidiously, and patients can have single or multiple episodic attacks, or persistent disease activity. An acute and severe onset of myositis may predict a particularly difficult course with severe, persistent, unresponsive disease. Any patient with an unexpectedly severe or perplexing clinical course, however, should be reevaluated for possible misdiagnosis or the development of another cause of muscle weakness. Although the patient and physician often focus on skeletal muscle involvement in these conditions, it is important to remember that the IIM are systemic connective tissue diseases with frequent extraskeletal manifestations. Patients may suffer from arthritis, a variety of skin disorders, and general symptoms such as fatigue, weight loss, Raynaud's phe-

TABLE 1. Associated Features of the Myositis Clinical and Serologic Groups

Group	Distinguishing Features	Disease Severity	Response to Therapy	Prognosis [Five yr Survival]
Clinical Groups				
Polymyositis	–none of the features below	variable	variable	moderate [80%]
Dermatomyositis	–heliotrope or Gottron's papules	mild to moderate	good to moderate	moderate [85%]
Connective tissue myositis	–overlap with other connective tissue diseases	mild	excellent	good [90%]
Cancer-associated myositis	–cancer diagnosed within 2 yr of IIM	variable	moderate to poor	poor, secondary to cancer [60%]
Juvenile myositis	–onset before 18 years of age –subcutaneous calcifications –gastrointestinal vasculitis	variable	variable	good [> 95%]
Inclusion body myositis	–insidious onset, distal weakness, atrophy, poor response to therapy	mild, progressive	poor	few deaths, but significant morbidity
Serologic Groups				
Anti-Synthetases	–acute onset, often in first half of the year –interstitial lung disease, fever, dyspnea on exertion, arthritis, mechanics hands, Raynaud's phenomena	moderate to severe	moderate, but flares with taper	poor [75%]
Anti-SRP [Signal Recognition Particle]	–very acute onset, often in the fall in Black females –palpitations, cardiac disease, severe weakness –no rash [clinically PM]	severe	poor	very poor [30%]
Anti-Mi-2	–Classic DM –"V" and "shawl sign" rashes, cuticular overgrowth	mild to moderate	good	good [> 95%]

nomenon, or fever. The gastrointestinal, cardiac, or pulmonary systems may also be involved which can both complicate therapy and adversely affect prognosis (1).

Clinical symptoms vary widely and often change over the course of the illness. Common signs and symptoms include: fatigue, muscle pain, atrophy, arthralgia and arthritis, rashes of many types, shortness of breath, dysphagia, edema, Raynaud's phenomenon, subcutaneous nodules and calcifications, dysphonia, fever, gastrointestinal pain, and weight loss. These findings appear to differ in the different clinical and serologic groups [Table 2].

THERAPY

General Considerations

The therapy of myositis has been poorly studied due to the rarity and heterogeneity of IIM. The goals of therapy are to eliminate inflammation in muscle and other involved tissues [induce remission] and to regain as much function as possible through physical therapy and rehabilitation. Although some children with myositis may have a monocyclic disease course and their disease may resolve easily with treatment, many adults require multiple courses of chronic therapy, and in some individuals disease activity cannot be controlled despite aggressive use of multiple agents (6,7). Because the clinical and serologic groups differ in the rapidity of myositis onset, severity of disease, responses to therapy, and clinical course, this information can be useful in deciding how quickly and aggressively to initiate treatment and how to alter subsequent therapy. A general problem in management has been the relative inability to predict responses to therapy and prognosis in individual myositis patients. Certain features, however, do appear to be useful in predicting prognosis among IIM groups [Table 3]. These include clinical and serologic group, delay from disease onset to treatment, severe myositis, and cardiac or pulmonary involvement. Patients with poor prognostic factors may benefit from earlier more aggressive therapy, although more study is needed in this area. To date, a scientifically-supported general scheme or flow diagram that would guide the therapy of all myositis patients has not been possible and today treatment needs to be individualized based upon the severity of disease, prognostic factors, and risk factors for adverse

TABLE 2. Frequencies [percent] of Selected Signs and Symptoms in the Major Myositis Clinical and Serologic Groups*

Sign/Symptom	All IIM	PM	DM	IBM	Synthetase	SRP	Mi-2
Fever	37	40	46	4	**87**	0	10
Raynaud's	35	37	40	4	**62**	29	30
Myalgias	60	68	71	26	84	**100**	60
Arthritis	47	54	55	9	**94**	0	20
Asymmetric weakness	14	10	4	**61**	4	0	0
Muscle atrophy	20	17	3	**96**	4	14	0
Falling	20	17	1	**96**	4	33	0
Dyspnea on exertion	51	**67**	59	9	94	43	50
Pulmonary fibrosis	29	40	37	0	**89**	0	0
Mechanic's hands	22	30	33	0	**71**	14	10
Gottron's papules or Heliotrope rash	45	0	**100**	0	40	0	**100**
Cuticular overgrowth	14	2	**30**	0	7	0	**100**
V-sign rash	17	0	**36**	0	15	0	**100**
Shawl-sign rash	10	0	22	0	7	0	**56**
Carpal tunnel	23	27	35	4	**49**	20	**56**

*Information from (5). Abbreviations: IIM, idiopathic inflammatory myopathies; PM, polymyositis; DM, dermatomyositis; IBM, inclusion body myositis; Synthetase, anti-synthetase autoantibody group; SRP, anti-signal recognition particle autoantibody group; Mi-2, anti-Mi-2 autoantibody group. Bolded numbers represent significantly higher frequencies [over-represented] compared to frequencies in one or more of the other groups listed.

TABLE 3. Poor Prognostic Factors in the Idiopathic Inflammatory Myopathies*

Poor Prognostic Category	Comments
Based upon Demographics:	
Black [versus white] race	May be related to socioeconomic factors and access to medical care as well as genetic differences
Old [versus young]	Repeatedly described in a number of studies
Female [versus male] gender	Not confirmed as a poor prognostic factor in some studies
Based upon Sign-Symptom Complex:	
Fever	May be related to being a component of the anti-synthetase syndrome
Severe myositis	May be related to the anti-SRP syndrome
Dysphagia	Possibly related to severe myositis
Pulmonary involvement	Also is a feature of the anti-synthetase syndrome
Cardiac involvement	A feature of the anti-SRP syndrome
Delay to diagnosis and therapy	Supported by many studies
Failure to induce complete remission	A feature of both the anti-synthetase and anti-SRP syndromes
Based upon Clinicopathologic Group:	
Polymyositis versus dermatomyositis	Possibly related to more severe myositis
Cancer-associated myositis	Most deaths from cancer rather than myositis
Inclusion body myositis	Little mortality but high morbidity
Based upon Serologic Group:	
Anti-synthetase autoantibodies	Possibly related to persistent myositis and pulmonary involvement
Anti-signal recognition particle autoantibodies	Possibly related to severe persistent myositis and cardiac involvement

* Information from (13,1).

effects of therapy in each patient. The current therapies reported to be possibly beneficial in some myositis groups are listed in Table 4.

Assessment of Disease Activity and Damage

Current therapies accepted as efficacious for the IIM have generally not been identified through randomized, controlled trials. Part of the reason for this has been the lack of validated ways to assess and distinguish disease activity [evidence of active inflammation that may benefit from anti-inflammatory treatment] from disease damage [permanent scarring or fibrosis that cannot be treated with an anti-inflammatory]. The assessment of myositis patient outcomes has not been standardized, and multiple outcome measures have been used in previous trials. Many of the previously used endpoints have been uni-dimensional, focusing exclusively on improvement in muscle strength in these systemic rheumatic diseases. To standardize the conduct and reporting of adult and juvenile myositis clinical studies and enhance the identification of effective therapeutic agents, an international group of more than 100 adult and pediatric rheumatologists, neurologists, dermatologists, physiatrists, and statisticians, known as the International Myositis Assessment and Clinical Studies Group [IMACS], has been formed. Through the use of Delphi and nominal group techniques to derive consensus, IMACS has proposed a core set of outcome measures for inclusion in all IIM trials, defined the degree of change in each core set measure that is clinically meaningful and has developed preliminary definitions of disease improvement, remission, and flare (8,9).

While IMACS has suggested six core set measures to evaluate disease in clinical trials [patient global assessment, physician global assessment, muscle strength, physical function, muscle enzymes, and extra-muscular activity assessment], these may not be user friendly in clinical practice. Most clinicians simply use global impressions, muscle strength, and enzymes as primary guides for therapy in their practices. Although serum creatine kinase [CK] levels correlate well with levels of the other myositis-associated enzymes [aldolase, LDH, AST/SGOT, ALT/SGPT], these enzymes do not accurately reflect disease activity in all patients, and do not correlate well with the degree of weakness, rash, and other extramuscular manifestations, or inflammation on biopsy in some patients. This may be due to circulating inhibitors of CK activity, the focal nature of the inflammation, the effects of prior episodes of myositis on residual strength, the concurrent development of another cause of muscle weakness, and differences in rates of change with time among these factors. Creatine kinase levels, for example, often rise a few weeks to months before myositis flares are clinically evident, and likewise, often decrease before clinical improvement.

TABLE 4. Possible Therapeutic Options for the Idiopathic Inflammatory Myopathies*

Agent	Myositis Subgroups Reported	Clinical Experience and Comments
Corticosteroids	All	Primary therapy for all forms of IIM; retrospective case series with historic controls suggest decreased mortality and less morbidity in PM, DM and JDM with oral or IV therapy
Methotrexate	All	Case reports and case series suggest improvement in muscle and skin in all myositis groups
Azathioprine	All	Positive case reports and 1 controlled trial in PM/DM suggest benefit
Methotrexate plus Azathioprine	PM, DM, IBM	Some evidence for efficacy in PM and DM in randomized cross over studies
Hydroxychloroquine sulfate	DM, JDM	Case reports and series suggest improvement in some myositis symptoms and rash
IVIG	All	Double-blind, placebo-controlled trial in DM shows good short term benefit; case series and open studies in JDM and PM suggest some benefit; IBM controlled studies do not show much benefit
Cyclophosphamide	PM, DM, JDM	Positive case reports and series; one negative open label study in PM and DM; possibly most useful as IV therapy in myositis pts with lung disease or vasculitis
Cyclosporin	PM, DM, JDM	Positive case reports and series
Tacrolimus	PM, DM	Small open label study showed good responses in pts with anti-Jo-1 and anti-SRP autoantibodies
Mycophenolate mofetil	PM, DM, JDM	Positive case reports and series
Anti-TNF alpha agents**	All	Open label case reports and series are more positive in DM and JDM than other groups; studies ongoing
Eculizumab [anti-C5 Mab]**	DM	Randomized, double-blind, placebo-controlled Phase 1 trial [N = 12] showed safety but little efficacy
Rituximab [anti-CD20 Mab]**	DM, JDM	Phase 1, open label, dose escalation trial ongoing with preliminary positive findings
Autologous stem cell therapy**	Anti-Jo-1+, PM, JDM	Case reports describe early response but late deaths in 2 PM pts, but good response in 1 JDM case; trials ongoing
Beta-Interferon**	IBM	Phase 1 randomized, placebo-controlled trial [N = 30] completed with some response; new trial ongoing

*Information from (12,14,15,7,16). Abbreviations: per Table 2; JDM, juvenile dermatomyositis; IVIG, intravenous immunoglobulin; anti-Jo-1, autoantibodies to Jo-1 antigen [histidyl-tRNA synthetase] present; pts, patients; CK, creatine kinase; TNF, tumor necrosis factor; Mab, monoclonal antibody.

** Agents with little experience or evidence of efficacy and that are currently undergoing study in clinical trials.

Corticosteroids

Corticosteroids remain the primary first line therapy for myositis, although in cases with poor prognostic features, additional immunosuppressives are often used from the beginning of disease. Important factors in achieving corticosteroid responses, in addition to the clinical and autoantibody group of the patient, are the adequacy of the initial dose [1-2 mg/kg/d], continuation of prednisone until or after the serum CK becomes normal, and a slow rate of prednisone tapering which averages 10 mg/month [about 25 percent of the existing dose per month]. Common errors in the use of corticosteroids in myositis include too rapid a taper before adequate clinical response and excessively high doses in the elderly and those with IBM. The roles of intravenous bolus corticosteroids and alternate day initial therapy remain unclear.

Other Management Issues and Approaches

Oral methotrexate and azathioprine remain the primary therapeutic options for corticosteroid-resistant patients. One study suggests that methotrexate may be superior to azathioprine, especially in men and patients with antisynthetase autoantibodies (10). In most of the other subgroups the choice of which of these two drugs to use is primarily determined by the individual risk factors of each patient. Intravenous gammaglobulin, cyclophosphamide, cyclosporin A, or combinations of cytotoxics may be beneficial in some subgroups of myositis patients and all warrant further evaluation. Pulse cyclophosphamide may be useful in the treatment of pulmonary fibrosis or vasculitis associated with IIM, especially in the context of the antisynthetase syndrome. Plasma exchange or leukapheresis do not appear to benefit steroid-resistant patients not taking cytotoxics as shown by a double-blinded sham-controlled trial. The extramuscular systemic manifestations of IIM can be difficult to treat. With the exception of the use of topical corticosteroids, hydroxychloroquine, and sunscreens for the treatment of the rash of dermatomyositis, no specific treatment has been definitively shown to benefit the systemic manifestations of the IIM.

Rehabilitation and physical therapy are often overlooked or underutilized in the management of myositis. These approaches are very important in maintaining range of motion and preventing contractures during active disease and exercise probably improves strength and endurance when initiated in a graded way during disease remission.

Some inclusion body myositis patients, particularly those with CKs greater than 1000 U/l and evidence of inflammation on muscle biopsy, may benefit from corticosteroid and cytotoxic therapy in terms of improvement in function or slowing the rate of progression of disease (11). Severe progressive dysphagia unresponsive to chemotherapy may benefit from cricopharyngeal myotomy.

Case reports and series suggest that targeted biologic agents, including monoclonal antibodies or fusion proteins directed at TNF-alpha, B cells or complement, as well as autologous stem cell approaches, might be beneficial and research is ongoing in this area (12).

CONCLUSION

Myositis patients present in a wide variety of ways and can sometimes be challenging to diagnose. It is important to remember the systemic nature of these syndromes and to fully evaluate patients for possible extramuscular manifestations. The specific signs and symptoms differ in the major IIM clinical and serologic groups and as such they can be useful guides for assessing possible organ system involvement.

Therapy for corticosteroid-resistant patients is poorly studied but includes cytotoxic agents and other immunomodulatory approaches. Dividing myositis patients into clinical and serologic groups results in subsets with different responses to therapy and different prognoses. Therapy should be individualized on the basis of disease severity, prognostic factors, and risks for side effects from the therapy itself. Patients in poorer prognostic groups [those with severe myositis, cardiopulmonary disease associated with myositis, the clinical group polymyositis, or the serologic groups with anti-synthetase or anti-SRP autoantibodies] should be considered for earlier and more aggressive therapy. The use of serology, immunopathology, and immunogenetics–as well as environmental exposures–to further subset the IIM, may define even more homogeneous groups. Proposed core outcome disease assessment measures and international collaborations will help to standardize the conduct and reporting of studies and enhance the efficiency of future clinical trials. These approaches, together with dramatic strides in understanding the molecular immunopathologic abnormalities in the myositis syndromes, should lead to a more complete understanding of the etiology and pathogenesis and better treatments for these increasingly recognized syndromes. Although we must temper the early optimism that often accompanies positive case reports and other uncontrolled experiences when a new agent is introduced, it is likely that one or more biologic therapies summarized in this review will find a role in the armamentarium of physicians who treat myositis in the future. Novel biologic and cellular therapies–coupled with the recent establishment of international multidisciplinary consortia that are developing consensus on outcome measures and clinical trial design issues in IIM to increase the efficiency and comparability of trials–will likely play an increasing role in understanding the best management of myositis disease activity and damage and will hopefully result in safer and more effective treatments in the future.

REFERENCES

1. Miller, F. W.: Inflammatory Myopathies: Polymyositis, dermatomyositis, and related conditions. In *Arthritis and Allied Conditions, A Textbook of Rheumatology*, 14th Edition, Lippincott, Williams and Wilkins, Philadelphia, W. Koopman, editor. Chapter 78, 1562-1589 (volume 2).

2. Shamim, E. A. and Miller, F. W.: Familial Autoimmunity and the Idiopathic Inflammatory Myopathies. Curr. Rheumatol. Rep. 2:201-211, 2000.

3. Shamim, E. A., Rider, L. G., and Miller, F. W.: Update on the genetics of the idiopathic inflammatory myopathies. Curr. Opin. Rheumatol. 12:482-491, 2000.

4. Miller, F. W.: Myositis-specific autoantibodies. Touchstones for understanding the inflammatory myopathies. Journal of the American Medical Association 270:1846-1849, 1993.

5. Love, L. A., Leff, R. L., Fraser, D. D., Targoff, I. N., Dalakas, M., Plotz, P. H., and Miller, F. W.: A new approach to the classification of idiopathic inflammatory myopathy: Myositis-specific autoantibodies define useful homogeneous patient groups. Medicine (Baltimore) 70:360-374, 1991.

6. Oddis, C. V.: Idiopathic inflammatory myopathy: Management and prognosis. Rheum. Dis. Clin. North Am. 28:979-1001, 2002.

7. Amato, A. A. and Griggs, R. C.: Treatment of idiopathic inflammatory myopathies. Curr. Opin. Neurol. 16:569-575, 2003.

8. Miller, F. W., Rider, L. G., Chung, Y. L., Cooper, R., Danko, K., Farewell, V., Lundberg, I., Morrison, C., Oakley, L., Oakley, I., Pilkington, C., Vencovsky, J., Vincent, K., Scott, D. L., and Isenberg, D. A.: Proposed preliminary core set measures for disease outcome assessment in adult and juvenile idiopathic inflammatory myopathies. Rheumatology (Oxford) 40:1262-1273, 2001.

9. Rider, L. G., Giannini, E. H., Harris-Love, M., Joe, G., Isenberg, D., Pilkington, C., Lachenbruch, P.

A., and Miller, F. W.: Defining Clinical Improvement in Adult and Juvenile Myositis. Journal of Rheumatology 30:603-617, 2003.

10. Joffe, M. M., Love, L. A., Leff, R. L., Fraser, D. D., Targoff, I. N., Hicks, J. E., Plotz, P. H., and Miller, F. W.: Drug therapy of the idiopathic inflammatory myopathies: Predictors of response to prednisone, azathioprine, and methotrexate and a comparison of their efficacy. Am. J. Med. 94:379-387, 1993.

11. Leff, R. L., Miller, F. W., Hicks, J. E., Fraser, D. D., and Plotz, P. H.: The treatment of inclusion body myositis: A retrospective review and a randomized, prospective trial of immunosuppressive therapy. Medicine 7233:225-235, 1993.

12. Miller, F. W.: Myositis. In *Targeted Therapies in Rheumatology*. Martin Dunitz, London. Chapter 36, 603-620. Edited by J.S. Smolen and P.E. Lipsky, 2003.

13. Miller, F. W.: Classification and prognosis of inflammatory muscle disease. Rheum. Dis. Clin. North. Am. 20:811-826, 1994.

14. Oddis, C. V.: Idiopathic inflammatory myopathy: Management and prognosis. Rheum. Dis. Clin. North Am. 28:979-1001, 2002.

15. Oddis, C. V.: Idiopathic inflammatory myopathies: A treatment update. Curr. Rheumatol. Rep. 5:431-436, 2003.

16. Rider, L. G. and Miller, F. W.: Idiopathic inflammatory muscle disease: Clinical aspects. Baillieres Best. Pract. Res. Clin. Rheumatol. 14:37-54, 2000.

Idiopathic Low Back Pain:
Classification and Differential Diagnosis

Bente Danneskiold-Samsøe
Else Marie Bartels

SUMMARY. Objectives: To present a contemporary view of the epidemiology, classification, and differential diagnosis of low back pain.

Findings: With age, the normal back will exhibit visible morphological changes. Thus, idiopathic low back pain cannot be directly related to the morphological picture, but is influenced by many factors related to ligaments, discs, muscles and nerves. Idiopathic low back pain is experienced in about two-thirds of the population over their life time and about half of the adult population will suffer from back pain at some time during a 12 months period. The cost to society for work absenteeism related to back pain is very high. There are a variety of systems for classifying back pain which do not always overlap, and which have different aims. The process of diagnosing back pain consists of clinical examination, various types of imaging, and laboratory tests. Imaging methods have improved greatly. For example, imaging can identify disc related problems, so patients with those lesions can be excluded from the idiopathic low back pain group. Despite improved methods, however, it is usually difficult to specify the cause of the low back pain, and it is still impossible to accurately perceive its severity.

Conclusions: Although acute back pain is often viewed as a benign and reversible condition, it can develop into a chronic condition if not correctly diagnosed and treated accordingly. *[Article copies available for a fee from The Haworth Document Delivery Service: 1-800-HAWORTH. E-mail address: <docdelivery@haworthpress.com> Website: <http://www.HaworthPress.com> © 2004 by The Haworth Press, Inc. All rights reserved.]*

KEYWORDS. Idiopathic low back pain, myofascial pain, fibromyalgia, muscle fatigue, pelvic pain

INTRODUCTION

The definition of low back pain is usually pain, muscle tension or stiffness localized below the costal margin and above the inferior gluteal folds, with or without sciatica. Furthermore, low back pain is classified as being specific or non-specific. When a specific pathophysiological mechanism causes low back pain, such as hernia nuclei pulposi, inflammation,

Bente Danneskiold-Samsøe, MD, DMSc, is Professor and Director, The Parker Institute, H. S. Frederiksberg Hospital, Nordre Fasanvej 57, 2000 Frederiksberg, Denmark [E-mail: bente.danneskiold@fh.hosp.dk].

Else Marie Bartels, PhD, DSc, is Senior Researcher, The Danish National Library of Science and Medicine, Nørre Allé 49, 2200 Copenhagen N, Denmark [E-mail: emb@dnlb.dk].

[Haworth co-indexing entry note]: "Idiopathic Low Back Pain: Classification and Differential Diagnosis." Danneskiold-Samsøe, Bente, and Else Marie Bartels. Co-published simultaneously in *Journal of Musculoskeletal Pain* [The Haworth Medical Press, an imprint of The Haworth Press, Inc.] Vol. 12, No. 3/4, 2004, pp. 93-99; and: *Soft Tissue Pain Syndromes: Clinical Diagnosis and Pathogenesis* [ed: Dieter E. Pongratz, Siegfried Mense, and Michael Spaeth] The Haworth Medical Press, an imprint of The Haworth Press, Inc., 2004, pp. 93-99. Single or multiple copies of this article are available for a fee from The Haworth Document Delivery Service [1-800-HAWORTH, 9:00 a.m. - 5:00 p.m. [EST]. E-mail address: docdelivery@haworthpress.com].

fractures, or tumor, we talk about specific low back pain, whereas non-specific low back pain [LBP] is characterized by pain of unknown origin, and of all patients with low back pain, the idiopathic LBP account for approximately 90 percent. The prognosis for these patients is excellent in regards to returning to work. Ninety percent return to work within six weeks. For about four percent of low back-pain sufferers, the recovery takes more than three months, and this group of patients accounts for around 75 percent of the socio-economical costs of LBP (1,2). Less than half of the low back-pain patients who have been off work for six months will return to work, but after being unable to work for two years, the chance of returning to work is non-existing (3). The low back-pain impact on disability and further on workability is obvious. An illustration of this is that one percent of the United States population is chronically disabled, and one percent is temporarily disabled, due to LBP.

In industrialized countries the prevalence, associated morbidity, and socio-economic cost of low back pain, directly and indirectly, are therefore well-documented to be high (4). The present situation is that although several studies have implicated some risk factors for LBP, these only seem to have a small or moderate effect (5-7). According to recent epidemiological studies, low back pain cannot be categorized as either acute or chronic, since there are fluctuations over time regarding onsets and exacerbations. Furthermore, low back pain may develop into a widespread pain situation. This may then lead to a diagnosis of fibromyalgia syndrome [FMS] instead of being perceived as isolated regional pain with a diagnosis of myofascial pain syndrome.

Although several studies have identified many individual, psychosocial, and occupational risk factors causing onset of low back pain and increased risk of chronic disability, no single factor seems to have a strong impact. Therefore, scientific studies addressing effects of primary and secondary prevention are still very much needed.

Successful management of low back pain requires that the treatment be specifically directed towards the pain-producing structures. Patients with low-back problems usually complain of both pain and disability. It is often as-sumed that the pain causes the disability, and if the pain condition is treated, the disability disappears. Unfortunately, this is not often the case, despite successful pain management. The reason is, of course, fundamental. There is not a simple relationship between pain experience and cause of disability, and failure to distinguish between pain and disability does have a major impact on the management of LBP. In order to reach a diagnosis of as high specificity as possible, one has to correlate a detailed clinical history and a thorough physical examination with radiographic investigations (8).

Clearly defined clinical guidelines are important, and depending on the referral level, they may differ for the general practitioner and a specialist of LBP in rheumatology, neurosurgery, or neurology. Particularly, when low back pain becomes a chronic condition, the psychological aspects must be taken into account in the treatment and management of the patient.

EPIDEMIOLOGIC FEATURES AND GENETIC INFLUENCES

The epidemiological concepts important when looking at the occurrence of low back pain are incidence, point prevalence, period prevalence, and lifetime prevalence (9).

> *Incidence* is the proportion of the population at issue that experiences low back pain for the first time in a particular time period.

> *Point prevalence* is the proportion of the population at issue that experiences low back pain at a particular point in time.

> *Period prevalence* is the proportion of the population at issue that experiences low back pain during a specific period.

> *Life-time prevalence* is the proportion of the population at issue that ever experienced an episode of low back pain during their life.

The life time incidence of LBP varies from 50 percent to over 80 percent with an average incidence of 60 percent (10). It is important when looking at incidence and prevalence values that these are obtained from the same specific population. In a United Kingdom LBP study (11), including more than 2,700 adults, the twelve months cumulative incidence of new LBP visits to the doctor was around four percent. Those with a previous history of back pain doubled the rate of episodes. Furthermore, patients appearing with widespread pain also had a much higher incidence of LBP in the past when compared to those with none. Also, the incidence of LBP was higher in men than in women, and the incidence was highest in the age group 25 to 64 years, the age group of working life.

Several studies have reported life-time prevalence data for LBP, and it ranges over a wide span [49 percent-70 percent], whereas point-prevalence studies [only a smaller number of studies] report point prevalence to be in the range of 12 percent-30 percent, and the period-prevalence studies show this to be in the range of 25 percent-42 percent (10).

There is, apart from the above, also a strong genetic influence both on disc degeneration and tendency towards psychological distress, as shown in studies of adult female twins (12).

RISK FACTORS

From an occupational point of view, LBP appears to be associated with heavy physical work, including lifting, bending, twisting, static work postures with long-term sitting, whole-body vibration, job dissatisfaction, and significant obesity. Also individual factors seem to play a role such as age, physical fitness, strength of back and abdominal muscles, and smoking. Psychosocial factors such as stress, anxiety, cognitive functioning, and pain behavior have been mentioned as well (13-17). Some predictors for chronicity of LBP are obesity, low educational level, high levels of pain and disability, distress, somatisation, and job requirement of lifting for around three-quarters of the working day.

PATHOLOGICAL FEATURES

Pathological changes may take place in different structures of the anatomical elements of the back, giving increasing pain from different tissues like bone, ligaments, joints, muscles, nerves, and connective tissue. The upper lumbar spine may be predisposed to compression of neural tissue within the central spinal canal, lateral recess, and foraminal areas. The intervertebral disc, posterior longitudinal ligament, zygapophyseal joint capsule, and ligamentum flavum define the spinal canal. Bone and soft tissue structures create these boundaries of the canal, and the relative contributions of these structures differ at different levels. The lateral recess comprises the lateral part of the canal and is found between the articular process posteriorly and the vertebral body anteriorly. Nerve roots run through the recess and further through the intervertebral foramen. It is obvious that the lumbar roots are in danger of excess pressure, especially when hypertrophic changes in both bone and soft tissue develop. Low back pain may, however, not only be caused by mechanical stress or pressure, but is rather more complicated involving both biomechanical, biochemical, physiological, and immunological processes in interaction.

CLINICAL COURSE

Although the prognosis for back pain is good, taken into account that most patients recover within two-four weeks without functional deficits, and a total of 90 percent have recovered in 12 weeks, the clinical course is not as promising as it appears at first sight. For the last 10 percent of the patients, the recovery is unfortunately slow. Another problem is that recurrence of LBP within the year following the initial episode is very frequent [up to 50 percent].

CLINICAL DIAGNOSIS AND DIFFERENTIAL DIAGNOSIS

A successful clinical course depends on a precise diagnosis. The LBP patients with a specific diagnosis are easy to identify. It is, however, difficult to identify the origin of LBP precisely in a high proportion of cases because, even when the disease characteristics seem to point towards a given structure or area, the pain often remains non-specific. The focus of medical attention has mainly been centred around trapped nerves, disc failure or damage, or bone defects, while no or little attention has been left to the soft tissue area where the stimulus for the pain sensation may have its origin.

It is a great challenge to examine LBP patients. During recent years, several clinical guidelines for diagnosing LBP have been published (18-22). All of these involve assessing risk of malignancy or severe infections, disc prolapse, spinal stenosis, and cauda equina syndrome. Lumbar disc diseases are examined with magnetic resonance imaging [MRI] as well (23) and may be visualized by discography (24), but this method may carry some risk when not performed with great skill.

Mechanical back pain and the facet joint syndrome are evoked by movement, usually by backward extension and rotation, where the facet joints are concerned. Facet joint pain is believed to evolve from repeated stretching, strain or entrapment of a fold of synovial membrane in the capsule, which surrounds the joint. Magnetic resonance imaging and/or computerized tomography [CT] scan may also here be useful diagnostically. A facet-joint nerve blocking is another important aid in this diagnosis (25,26). Sacroiliac joint syndromes may be related to inflammatory diseases, but may also be related to pregnancy (27,28). Rare cases of LBP are sacral stress fractures (29) and diffuse idiopathic skeletal hyperostosis (30), and these cases may give rise to differential diagnostic problems. This is also the case for coccygodynia (31,32). A measurement of intradiscal pressure is today another possibility in patients with ongoing back problems to exclude/include stress of the measured disc area (33).

Imaging

New imaging methods like MRI, CT-scanning and ultrasound have given a set of wonderful tools with which one may examine LBP patients, and especially MRI is now widely used and is a great advance when diagnosing LBP (34,35). Despite this, it is still very important not to rely completely on these methods, but to remember the basic clinical skills when assessing the LBP patients, in case there might be other causes than the changes seen on the scan.

A specific diagnosis is often associated with traumatic injury, neoplasm, infection, or neurological deficit. A non-specific diagnosis will mostly present itself with a clinical picture of pain only, and by examination the findings are sparse, although the symptoms are manifold. Even professionals do not always routinely examine for myofascial abnormalities which are universally present and are the most frequent source of the painful state, when looking at LBP patients. New techniques for soft tissue measurements and further scientific developments of already existing objective electromyographic fatigue test are much needed and may hopefully be developed in this area (36,37). Specially designed eccentric and isokinetic muscle strength examinations (38,39) and experimental gait analysis in LBP are other possible assessment methods (40).

Classification of Non-Specific Low Back Pain

Malterud and Hollnagel (41) in 1997 defined classification systems for sorting complex elements of reality into reasonable and logical entities. The medical classification system deals with disease location expressed as diagnosis. The main purpose of classification in diagnosing is to find the causes, to predict the outcome, and to determine a specific treatment of a disease.

Idiopathic LBP with an unspecific diagnosis makes decisions of choice of treatment difficult, since there are many available possibilities. The need of classification systems to handle a further and more precise diagnosis of LBP is obvious. The heterogeneity of both symptoms and appearance of the patients with idiopathic LBP and the wide variety of treatment modalities given to these patients is an enormous problem. This is probably the reason for the very limited number of studies of properly designed research in the area, and thereby the lack of conclusions on the outcome of the different types of treatment of idiopathic LBP. We have to acknowledge that further testing of validity of categories to identify symptomatic anatomical structures in the lower back is very much needed. As it stands today, selected idiopathic LBP patients may overlap with or be composed of other patient groups from the defined pain syndromes such as myofascial pain, FMS, hypermobility, coccodynia, as well as patients with facet joint and sacroiliac problems, as illustrated in Figures 1 and 2.

A recent study dealing with chronic LBP and FMS (42) has shown that the prevalence of primary and secondary FMS in patients with spinal pain is rather low [12 percent]. It is on the other hand concluded that FMS may be the cause of low back pain in patients, who may be unaware of pain in other areas in the musculoskeletal system or have problems defining the more unspecific pain sensations, while back pain is something easy to comprehend. In a retrospective study, the frequency of transition of chronic LBP to FMS was 25 percent and predictive parameters for the chance of LBP developing into FMS were sex and postural disorders

FIGURE 1. The model shows how the diagnosis may be created of symptoms and objective findings. When the diagnosis is established by specific symptoms and examinations it becomes precise.

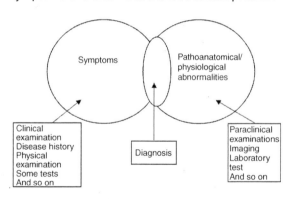

FIGURE 2. Idiopathic LBP illustrated by the large box may be comprised of some smaller boxes with other syndromes, even some we do not yet know.

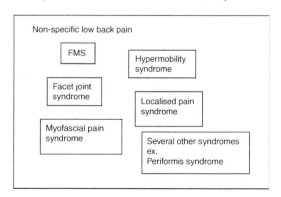

such as scoliosis (43). Another finding is that there is a clear reduction of the mobility of the spine when comparing FMS patients to normal controls (44). Based on present knowledge it therefore seems likely that the spine plays a major role in the development of FMS. It may be hypothesised that chronic local pain may develop via repeated mechanical irritation. This may take place in the small vertebral joints and/or ligaments in connections with these, and activations of nociceptors in these regions, perhaps combined with muscle spasms, will trigger a postural problem. The sensation of these stimuli may be associated with the release of inflammatory mediators, especially substance P, that cause pain. The further spread of pain may arise from both neural and muscular pathways in connection with further postural problems in an interaction between biomechanical, biochemical, physiological, and immunological factors. The result may be a generalization of pain, thereby bringing about the disease picture of FMS.

Pain and Low Back Problems

Clauw et al. (54) have shown that pain sensitivity is correlated with clinical status of individuals with chronic LBP. Although a pilot study, the data gives evidence for that a person's experimental pain threshold is associated with baseline functional status and pain in cases of chronic LBP.

The final experience of pain is situated in the brain and is the result of the various pain signals from the peripheral pain receptors. We are often able to locate the area where the pain is created but seldom the origin of this tissue pain. Referred pain is also a complication in diagnosing the site and origin of LBP. In a newly published study (46) there is shown evidence of augmented central pain processing in chronic idiopathic LBP as well as in FMS patients which may again speak for a closer investigation of the relationship between the two conditions and the origin of the pain experience and the disability of both diseases.

CONCLUSION

Today there are good diagnostic methods to define most types of LBP. We are, though, left with a group of unspecific LBP, which carry the risk of developing into chronic LBP. What is now needed is a concentrated effort to work out a set of usable and clear classification systems for this particular group of patients. When this group is well defined in detail, a more successful and specific treatment can be implemented, and guidelines for management of the idiopathic LBP patients can be decided based on controlled studies of well-defined patient groups.

Very little has been done in considering the impact of inflammation on LBP and chronic muscular pain. A perturbation of the immunological system caused by minor infections may cause an irritation of the soft tissue. With further irritations this may turn into a chronic pain condition. It may, therefore, be advisable to test idiopathic LBP patients for changes in the immunological parameters. It is important too to follow these patients over time, both in the acute phase and longitudinally in order to find the true cause and effect.

The development of the various imaging methods has been of great importance in diagnosing LBP more specifically. A further development of these methods will probably bring us many steps further. However, development of other types of new assessment methods for the less defined part of the idiopathic LBP patient group is very much needed, and research in this field must now have a high priority. This is especially crucial when it comes to the implementation.

Based on that even the LBP patients who are back at work and free of pain in four weeks after onset often experience reoccurrences of LBP, longitudinal studies following the patients both in the acute phases of LBP and in the periods between these are one of the most important areas of research in LBP, if successful treatment, and even more so, prevention can be applied.

REFERENCES

1. Nachemson AL: Instability of the lumbar spine. Pathology, treatment, and clinical evaluation. Neurosurg Clin N Am 24:785-790, 1991.

2. Nachemson AL: Spinal disorders. Overall impact on society and the need for orthopedic resources. Acta Orthop Scand Suppl 241:17-22, 1991.

3. Waddel G: The Clinical Course of Back Pain. The Back Pain Revolution. Edinburgh: Churchill Livingstone, pp. 103-107, 1998.

4. Deyo RA, Weinstein JN: Low back pain. N Engl J Med 344(5):363-370, 2001.

5. Croft PR, Papageorgiou AC, Ferry S, Thomas E, Jayson MI, Silman AJ: Psychologic distress and low back pain. Evidence from a prospective study in the general population. Spine 20(24):2731-2737, 1995.

6. Croft PR, Macfarlane GJ, Papageorgiou AC, Thomas E, Silman AJ: Outcome of low back pain in general practice: A prospective study. BMJ 316(7141): 1356-1359, 1998.

7. Croft PR, Papageorgiou AC, Thomas E, Macfarlane GJ, Silman AJ: Short-term physical risk factors for new episodes of low back pain. Prospective evidence from the South Manchester Back Pain Study. Spine 24(15):1556-1561, 1999.

8. Bernard TN, Jr., Kirkaldy-Willis WH: Recognizing specific characteristics of nonspecific low back pain. Clin Orthop 217:266-280, 1987.

9. van Tulder M, Koes B, Bombardier C: Low back pain. Best Pract Res Clin Rheumatol 165:761-775, 2002.

10. Andersson GB: Low back pain. J Rehabil Res Dev: 344:ix, 1997.

11. Papageorgiou AC, Croft PR, Thomas E, Ferry S, Jayson MI, Silman AJ: Influence of previous pain experience on the episode incidence of low back pain: Results from the South Manchester Back Pain Study. Pain 66(2-3):181-185, 1996.

12. MacGregor AJ, Andrew T, Sambrook PN, Spector TD: Structural, psychological, and genetic influences on low back and neck pain: A study of adult female twins. Arthritis Rheum 51(2):160-167, 2004.

13. Waxman R, Tennant A, Helliwell P: A prospective follow-up study of low back pain in the community. Spine 25(16):2085-2090, 2000.

14. Deyo RA, Andersson G, Bombardier C, Cherkin DC, Keller RB, Lee CK et al.: Outcome measures for studying patients with low back pain. Spine 19 (Suppl 18):2032S-2036S, 1994.

15. Marras WS, Davis KG, Ferguson SA, Lucas BR, Gupta P: Spine loading characteristics of patients with low back pain compared with asymptomatic individuals. Spine 26(23):2566-2574, 2001.

16. Helewa A, Goldsmith C, Smythe HA: Inflammatory myopathy–Do we have adequate measures of the treatment response? J Rheumatol 21(9):1775, 1994.

17. Helewa A, Goldsmith CH, Lee P, Smythe HA, Forwell L: Does strengthening the abdominal muscles prevent low back pain–A randomized controlled trial. J Rheumatol 26(8):1808-1815, 1999.

18. Rosomoff HL, Rosomoff RS: Low back pain. Evaluation and management in the primary care setting. Med Clin North Am 83(3):643-662, 1999.

19. Davies M, Cassar-Pullicino VN: MRI of degenerative lumbar intervertebral disc disease. CME Radiology 31:3-10, 2002.

20. Jarvik JG: Imaging of adults with low back pain in the primary care setting. Neuroimaging Clin N Am 13(2):293-305, 2003.

21. Gulati P, Shikha D: Imaging in spinal disorders. JIMSA141:20-30, 2001.

22. Chin CT. Spine imaging. Semin Neurol 22(2): 205-220, 2002.

23. Carrino JA, Morrison WB: Imaging of lumbar degenerative disc disease. Seminars in Spine Surgery 154:361-383, 2003.

24. Ortiz AO, Johnson B: Discography. Tech Vasc Interv Radiol 54:207-216, 2002.

25. Mehta M, Parry CB: Mechanical back pain and the facet joint syndrome. Disabil Rehabil 16(1):2-12, 1994.

26. Helbig T, Lee CK: The lumbar facet syndrome. Spine 13(1):61-64, 1988.

27. Albert HB, Godskesen M, Westergaard JG: Incidence of four syndromes of pregnancy-related pelvic joint pain. Spine 27(24):2831-2834, 2002.

28. Damen L, Buyruk HM, Guler-Uysal F, Lotgering FK, Snijders CJ, Stam HJ: Pelvic pain during pregnancy is associated with asymmetric laxity of the sacroiliac joints. Acta Obstet Gynecol Scand 80(11):1019-1024, 2001.

29. Lin JT, Lane JM: Sacral stress fractures. J Womens Health Larchmt 12(9):879-888, 2003.

30. Belanger TA, Rowe DE: Diffuse idiopathic skeletal hyperostosis: Musculoskeletal manifestations. J Am Acad Orthop Surg 94:258-267, 2001.

31. Wray CC, Easom S, Hoskinson J: Coccydynia. Aetiology and tretment. J Bone Joint Surg Br 73(2): 335-338, 1991.

32. Maigne JY, Lagauche D, Doursounian L: Instability of the coccyx in coccydynia. J Bone Joint Surg Br 82(7):1038-1041, 2000.

33. Sato K, Kikuchi S, Yonezawa T: In vivo intradiscal pressure measurement in healthy individuals and in patients with ongoing back problems. Spine 24(23): 2468-2474, 1999.

34. Leonardi M, Simonetti L, Agati R: Neuroradiology of spine degenerative diseases. Best Pract Res Clin Rheumatol 16(1):59-87, 2002.

35. Longo M, Granata F, Ricciardi K, Gaeta M, Blandino A: Contrast-enhanced MR imaging with fat suppression in adult-onset septic spondylodiscitis. Eur Radiol 133:626-637, 2003.

36. Koumantakis GA, Arnall F, Cooper RG, Oldham JA: Paraspinal muscle EMG fatigue testing with two methods in healthy volunteers. Reliability in the context of clinical applications. Clin Biomech Bristol, Avon 163:263-266, 2001.

37. Sparto PJ, Parnianpour M, Barria EA, Jagadeesh JM: Wavelet analysis of electromyography for back muscle fatigue detection during isokinetic constant-torque exertions. Spine 24(17):1791-1798, 1999.

38. Huang QM, Thorstensson A: Trunk muscle strength in eccentric and concentric lateral flexion. Eur J Appl Physiol 83(6):573-577, 2000.

39. Shirado O, Ito T, Kaneda K, Strax TE: Concentric and eccentric strength of trunk muscles: Influence of test postures on strength and characteristics of patients with chronic low-back pain. Arch Phys Med Rehabil 76(7):604-611, 1995.

40. Arendt-Nielsen L, Graven-Nielsen T, Svarrer H, Svensson P: The influence of low back pain on muscle activity and coordination during gait: A clinical and experimental study. Pain 64(2):231-240, 1996.

41. Malterud K, Hollnagel H: The magic influence of classification systems in clinical practice. Scand J Prim Health Care 151:5-6, 1997.

42. Borenstein D: Prevalence and treatment outcome of primary and secondary fibromyalgia in patients with spinal pain. Spine 20(7):796-800, 1995.

43. Lapossy E, Maleitzke R, Hrycaj P, Mennet W, Muller W: The frequency of transition of chronic low back pain to fibromyalgia. Scand J Rheumatol 24(1): 29-33, 1995.

44. Muller W, Kelemen J, Stratz T: Spinal factors in the generation of fibromyalgia syndrome. Z Rheumatol 57 Suppl 2:36-42, 1998.

45 Clauw DJ, Williams D, Lauerman W, Dahlman M, Aslami A, Nachemson AL et al.: Pain sensitivity as a correlate of clinical status in individuals with chronic low back pain. Spine 24(19):2035-2041, 1999.

46. Giesecke T, Gracely RH, Grant MA, Nachemson A, Petzke F, Williams DA et al.: Evidence of augmented central pain processing in idiopathic chronic low back pain. Arthritis Rheum 50(2):613-623, 2004.

Central Nervous Sequelae of Local Muscle Pain

Siegfried Mense
U. Hoheisel

SUMMARY. Objectives: To give an overview of some of the events that occur in the spinal cord as a reaction to a painful lesion of a peripheral muscle and that may be of importance for the transition from acute to chronic muscle pain.

Findings: In rats with an experimental myositis, marked changes are visible in the connectivity of the dorsal horn within a few hours. One of these neuroplastic changes was reflected in an increase of the target area of the muscle nerve in the dorsal horn, i.e, the myositis-induced excitation in the spinal cord expanded. This expansion is the result of a sensitization of dorsal horn neurons that become hyperexcitable by the continuous input from the inflamed muscle. Receptors for glutamate and substance P are involved in this process. The nitric oxide-cyclic guanosine monophosphate axis appears to be responsible for the spontaneous pain in patients rather than for the hyperalgesia. Glial cells [e.g., astrocytes] show a strong reaction to chronic muscle lesions and synthesize agents that influence neurons.

Conclusions: The transition from acute to chronic muscle pain is assumed to consist of a series of processes that start with the muscle lesion. Functional changes in the spinal dorsal horn are fastest [e.g., opening of "silent synapses"], metabolic changes [e.g., in the NO-cGMP pathway] are slower. The slowest processes are morphologic alterations that fix the initially functional changes. It is generally assumed that any longer-lasting muscle lesion is associated with such central nervous alterations. The fact that not all patients with muscle lesions become chronic pain patients can be explained by the complexity of mechanisms involved [not all mechanisms are active in all patients]. Moreover, mechanisms that counteract the transition from acute to chronic pain also exist and vary in strength among patients [e.g., the degree of activity in antinociceptive pathways of the synthesis of the inhibitory factor FGF-2 by astrocytes]. Investigations in the near future are expected to yield many new insights regarding the role of glial cells in chronic pain. The importance of this cell system appears to be much greater than assumed in the past. *[Article copies available for a fee from The Haworth Document Delivery Service: 1-800-HAWORTH. E-mail address: <docdelivery@ haworthpress.com> Website: <http://www.HaworthPress.com> © 2004 by The Haworth Press, Inc. All rights reserved.]*

KEYWORDS. Central sensitization, nitric oxide, cyclic guanosine monophosphate, glial cells

Siegfried Mense, Prof. Dr. med., and U. Hoheisel, Dr. rer. nat., Research Assistant, are affiliated with Universität Heidelberg, Heidelberg, Germany.

Address correspondence to: Siegfried Mense, Prof. Dr. med., Institut für Anatomy und Zellbiologie III, Universität Heidelberg, Im Neuenheimer Feld 307, D-69120 Heidelberg, Germany [E-mail: mense@urz.uni-heidelberg.de].

[Haworth co-indexing entry note]: "Central Nervous Sequelae of Local Muscle Pain." Mense, Siegfried, and U. Hoheisel. Co-published simultaneously in *Journal of Musculoskeletal Pain* [The Haworth Medical Press, an imprint of The Haworth Press, Inc.] Vol. 12, No. 3/4, 2004, pp. 101-109; and: *Soft Tissue Pain Syndromes: Clinical Diagnosis and Pathogenesis* [ed: Dieter E. Pongratz, Siegfried Mense, and Michael Spaeth] The Haworth Medical Press, an imprint of The Haworth Press, Inc., 2004, pp. 101-109. Single or multiple copies of this article are available for a fee from The Haworth Document Delivery Service [1-800-HAWORTH, 9:00 a.m. - 5:00 p.m. [EST]. E-mail address: docdelivery@ haworthpress.com].

Available online at http://www.haworthpress.com/web/JMP
© 2004 by The Haworth Press, Inc. All rights reserved.
doi:10.1300/J094v12n03_15

MYOSITIS-INDUCED NEUROPLASTIC CHANGES IN THE SPINAL DORSAL HORN

Input from muscle nociceptors to the spinal cord or brain stem is known to be particularly effective to induce changes in the function, and later connectivity, of sensory dorsal horn neurons (1,2). In rats, such changes occur within a few hours after an experimental muscle lesion. In previous animal experiments of our group, the most prominent effect of an acute experimental inflammation [two to eight hour duration] of the gastrocnemius-soleus [GS] muscle was an expansion of the spinal input region of the GS muscle nerve [i.e., the population of dorsal horn neurons responding to electrical stimulation of the nerve grew larger] (2). This effect was most marked in the spinal segment L3, which under normal conditions receives only marginal input from the GS muscle. The most likely explanation for these changes is that the synaptic connections between muscle afferents and the neurons in L3 have become more efficient in myositis animals.

According to recent concepts of the transition from acute to chronic pain, the higher synaptic efficacy is due to hyperexcitability of the spinal neurons caused by the nociceptive input from the inflamed muscle [central sensitization] (3,4). Through this mechanism, formerly ineffective ["silent"] synapses in the border area of the GS input region may become effective. In patients, this hyperexcitability is likely to cause more pain in response to a noxious stimulus [i.e., hyperalgesia]. Central sensitization is considered one of the first steps in the transition from acute to chronic muscle pain.

At the molecular level, the following processes are assumed to occur in dorsal horn neurons when silent synapses become effective [Figure 1]. Normally, a nociceptive synapse in the spinal dorsal horn releases glutamate in response to a short noxious stimulus [e.g., a blow to the muscle]. Postsynaptically, glutamate opens the alpha-amino-3-hydroxyl-5-meth-

FIGURE 1. Transition from an ineffective [silent] to an effective synapse [simplified figure]. **A.** State before any strong nociceptive input. In the presynaptic ending of the afferent group IV fiber the neurotransmitter glutamate and the neuromodulator substance P [SP] are stored. On the postsynaptic side, the neurokinin receptor 1 [NK 1] for SP and two receptors for glutamate are shown: the alpha-amino-3-hydroxyl-5-methylisoxazole-proprionic acid/kainite [AMPA/KA] and the N-methyl-D-aspartate [NMDA] receptor. The NMDA receptor is permeable to Ca^{++} ions, but normally it is blocked by an Mg^{++} ion. Only after the Mg^{++} ion has been removed [e.g., by depolarization brought about by binding of SP to the NK 1 receptor] can glutamate open the NMDA channel. **B.** State after strong or long-lasting nociceptive input. Glutamate and SP have been released together, this opens the NMDA channel and Ca^{++} ions enter the postsynaptic cell. Ca^{++} activates intracellular enzymes that phosphorylate–transfer phosphate residues– to AMPA channels. The phosphorylated AMPA channels are better permeable to Na^+ ions, and the synapse becomes effective. For details, see text.

Resting state [silent synapse]   After strong noxious input

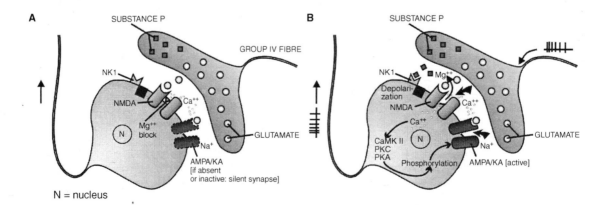

ylisoxazole-proprionic acid/kainite [AMPA/KA] ion channel and Na+-ions enter the cell. This causes a short excitation, and thereafter the cell returns to its normal state of excitability. Apparently, many central synapses have ineffective AMPA channels [with poor permeability for ions], or these channels are completely missing. Such synapses are ineffective or silent under normal conditions. Under pathophysiological circumstances [long-lasting or strong nociceptive input], glutamate and substance P [SP] are released together from the presynaptic ending of the muscle afferent fiber. The combined action of glutamate and SP opens postsynaptic N-methyl-D-aspartate [NMDA] channels through which Ca++-ions enter the dorsal horn neuron. Ca++-ions are second messengers that activate intracellular enzymes. One [out of many] effect of the enzymes is to phosphorylate existing ion channels in the membrane of the postsynaptic neuron. If an ineffective AMPA channel is phosphorylated, it becomes more effective [i.e., is better permeable for ions or opens for a longer period of time in response to a depolarization].

In the long run, the gene expression in the nucleus of the neuron also changes, which can lead to a de-novo synthesis of AMPA/KA ion channel proteins and others. The overall result of these processes is a sensitized neuron that is hyperexcitable by noxious and innocuous stimuli. In patients, the opening of silent synapses may cause spread and referral of muscle pain.

NEUROTRANSMITTERS INVOLVED IN CENTRAL SENSITIZATION

As outlined above, SP acting on neurokinin 1 [NK 1] receptors and glutamate acting on NMDA receptors are involved in the neuronal hyperexcitability and the lesion-induced expansion of the target area (5). In contrast, the background activity [i.e., neuronal activity in the absence of intentional stimulation] of the same dorsal horn neurons appears to depend strongly on the release of nitric oxide [NO] in the spinal cord (6). If the enzyme that synthesizes NO [nitric oxide synthase [NOS]] is blocked experimentally by intrathecal administration of N^G-nitro-L-arginine methyl ester [L-NAME], the background activity of nociceptive neurons

rises markedly. This suggests that normally NO is released continuously in the dorsal horn and inhibits the background discharge of nociceptive neurons. The background activity is of clinical importance because it is assumed to be responsible for spontaneous pain and dysesthesia in patients. The effects of NO are discussed controversially in the literature, with some regarding it as a pronociceptive and some as an antinociceptive agent. One possible explanation for this apparent discrepancy is that NO has antinociceptive properties at the spinal level and pronociceptive properties in supraspinal centers. This concept is supported by data obtained with interventions in the NO-cyclic guanosine monophosphate [cGMP] pathway [see below].

Patients with myositis complain of hyperalgesia, hyperesthesia, spontaneous pain, dysesthesia, and weakness (7,8). The above data suggest that the hyperalgesia is mediated by activation of NK 1 and NMDA receptors, whereas the spontaneous pain results from other processes [e.g., reduced spinal release of NO].

THE NITRIC OXIDE-CYCLIC GUANOSINE MONOPHOSPHATE [NO-CGMP] AXIS AS A FACTOR FOR CHRONIC MUSCLE PAIN

In the central nervous system, NO acts as a highly diffusible second messenger that is synthesized in a small subset of neurons, diffuses out of the cell right after synthesis and influences adjacent neurons or glial cells. Here, it activates the soluble form of the guanylyl cyclase and thus increases the synthesis of cyclic guanosine monophosphate [cGMP] (9), [Figure 2]. Both NO and cGMP have been shown to be involved in nociceptive processing (10-14). Spinally administered NO donors caused a depression of ongoing impulse [background] activity in spinal dorsal horn neurons (15,16), and inhibition of the spinal nitric oxide synthase led to an increase in background activity (16,17) of nociceptive neurons (17). Administration of 8-bromo-cGMP mimicked the effect of NO donors (15), indicating that cGMP is involved in the NO-induced reduction of impulse activity.

FIGURE 2. The nitric oxide-cGMP pathway. The scheme shows the blockers used and their target enzymes. Enzymes: Nitric oxide [NO] synthase catalyses the formation of NO from L-arginine, NO activates the soluble guanylyl cyclase which in turn catalyses the formation of cyclic guanosine monophosphate [cGMP] from guanosine triphosphate [GTP]. At the end of the cascade, the cGMP-specific phosphodiesterase type 5 hydrolyses cGMP to 5'-GMP. Inhibitors: 1. N^G-nitro-L-arginine methyl ester [L-NAME], a blocker of the NO synthase [leads to a reduction of NO level]. 2. 1H-[1,2,4]oxadiazolo [4,3-a]quinoxalin-1-one [ODQ], a selective blocker of the NO-sensitive guanylyl cyclase [leads to a reduction of cGMP level]. 3. Sildenafil, a selective blocker of the cGMP specific phosphodiesterase type 5 [leads to an increase of the cGMP level].

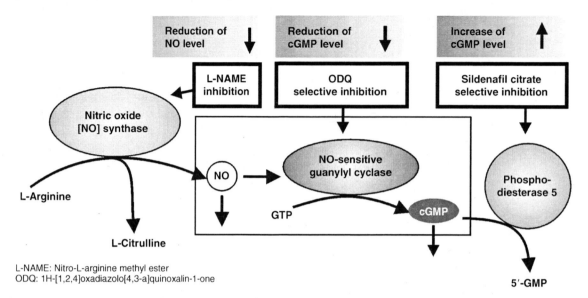

L-NAME: Nitro-L-arginine methyl ester
ODQ: 1H-[1,2,4]oxadiazolo[4,3-a]quinoxalin-1-one

A novel therapeutic substance that acts on the cGMP metabolism is sildenafil. The drug inhibits the degradation of cGMP by the enzyme phosphodiesterase 5 [Figure 2] and is used in the treatment of male erectile dysfunction (18). Recent clinical data show that following oral treatment with sildenafil some patients and healthy subjects complain of marked muscle pain mainly in the lower back (19,20). Apparently, sildenafil influences nociceptive processing by increasing spinal or supraspinal levels of cGMP.

In experiments on rats, our group tested the hypothesis that cGMP or NO have different actions at spinal or supraspinal levels (12). In these experiments, inhibitors of enzymes controlling the NO-cGMP synthesis were administered systemically, spinally, or supraspinally, and discharges of dorsal horn neurons were recorded at the lumbar level.

The following inhibitors of enzymes controlling the cGMP metabolism were used [Figure 2]: 1. L-NAME, a blocker of the NO synthesis. It indirectly lowers the cGMP level.

2. 1H-[1,2,4]oxadiazolo[4,3-a]quinoxalin-1-one [ODQ], a selective inhibitor of the NO-sensitive guanylyl cyclase, which lowers cGMP. 3. sildenafil citrate, a selective inhibitor of the cGMP specific phosphodiesterase type 5 that catalyses the hydrolysis of cGMP to guanosine monophosphate [GMP]. It increases the level of cGMP.

Systemic [i.v. or oral] administration of sildenafil caused a strong increase in the activity of lumbar dorsal horn neurons [Figure 3]. As such an activity at the lumbar level most probably is responsible for the low back pain of patients taking sildenafil, these data show that our animal model is suitable for studying the pain-inducing effects of sildenafil. The sildenafil-induced activity was not reduced when the exposed spinal cord was additionally superfused with ODQ to block cGMP synthesis locally in the dorsal horn. The ODQ data were the first indication that the pain-inducing effect of sildenafil was not due to a spinal action.

Intrathecal administration [local spinal superfusion]: The frequency of the neurons was

FIGURE 3. Impulse activity of a nociceptive dorsal horn neuron after intravenous injection of sildenafil. Upper panel: Original recording of the onset of the sildenafil-induced background activity. Lower panel: Histogram of the neuron's discharge frequency. The neuron had nociceptive properties with a receptive field in the deep tissues of the dorsum of the hind paw. It required noxious–subjectively painful–pressure stimulation [Nox. p.] for activation [Mod. p., moderate, innocuous pressure]. The duration of sildenafil injection is indicated by the filled bar underneath the histogram.

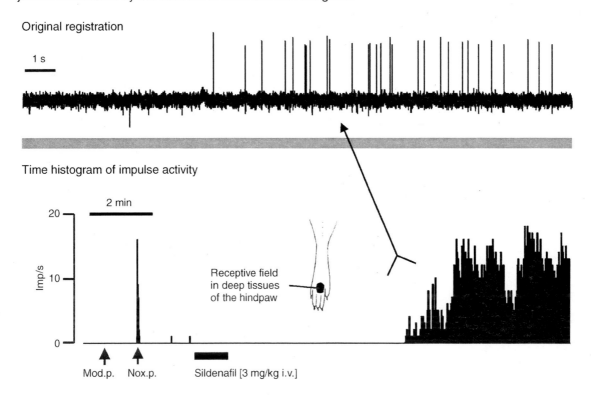

markedly increased by spinal ODQ and L-NAME superfusion [Figure 4A]. These data show that a block of the cGMP-synthesis in the dorsal horn–induced either by ODQ or L-NAME–is an excitatory stimulus for dorsal horn neurons. Sildenafil i.t. had no effect on the neurons.

Intracerebroventricular [i.c.v.] injections: In contrast to spinal sildenafil superfusion, injections of sildenafil into the third ventricle caused a strong increase of neuronal activity in the lumbar spinal cord [Figure 4B]. These data suggest that sildenafil has an effective site of action at the supraspinal level, and that following systemic administration the excitatory action of sildenafil on lumbar dorsal horn neurons is due to an action of the drug on supraspinal centers which in turn influence the lumbar neurons via descending modulating pathways. There are data indicating that sildenafil is able to cross the blood-brain barrier (21). Apparently, a *decrease* of cGMP in the spinal cord has

an excitatory action on nociceptive dorsal horn neurons, whereas at the supraspinal level, an *increase* of cGMP is excitatory for these neurons. The increase in background activity induced by sildenafil intra-cerebroventricularly occurred predominantly in nociceptive dorsal horn neurons. Following sildenafil treatment, the proportion of active neurons increased significantly in nociceptive but not in non-nociceptive dorsal horn neurons.

The excitatory effect of supraspinally injected sildenafil on lumbar neurons might be due to a depressing action of the increased cGMP level on descending inhibitory or a stimulating effect on excitatory descending tracts which led to an excitation of lumbar neurons (22). Besides the ventrolateral medulla, which is supposed to be the main origin of the tonic descending inhibition in anesthetized animals (23), various other supraspinal centers are known to contribute to the descending inhibi-

FIGURE 4. Impulse activity of dorsal horn neurons during local spinal superfusion and following intra-cerebroventricular injection of L-NAME, ODQ, and sildenafil. **A.** Experiments with spinal superfusion. Control [CSF, open bar], results from animals in which the spinal cord was superfused with CSF [artificial cerebrospinal fluid]; L-NAME [light grey bar], spinal superfusion with 100 µM L-NAME; ODQ [dark grey bar], spinal superfusion with 100 µM ODQ; Sildenafil [filled bars], spinal superfusion with 1 µM and 100 µM sildenafil, respectively. **B.** Experiments with intracerebroventricular injections into the third ventricle. The injection volume was 10 µl. ***, P < 0.001, difference between CSF and inhibitor.

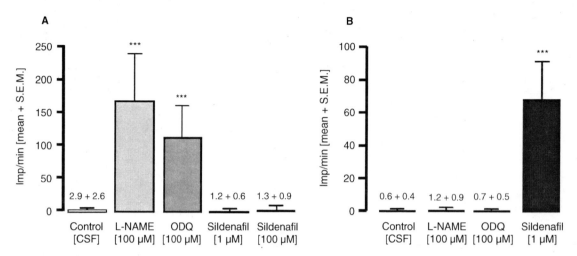

tion, e.g., periventricular grey, amygdala, and ventrobasal thalamus (22,24); for a review see (25).

As to the pain induced by sildenafil orally in patients, our data indicate that the low back pain is due to an action of sildenafil on supraspinal centers that excite nociceptive dorsal horn neurons via descending pain-modulating tracts.

OTHER FACTORS FOR THE TRANSITION FROM ACUTE TO CHRONIC PAIN

Recent data indicate that hyperexcitable neurons and chronic pain also can be induced through the mechanism of excitotoxicity (26). The concept of excitotoxicity states that a strong nociceptive input releases large amounts of SP and glutamate simultaneously. This leads to a maximal opening of all of the calcium-permeable ion channels. The postsynaptic cells are swamped with Ca^{++}, which activates all of the enzymes that are present in the cytoplasm. Among these enzymes are some that are dangerous for the cell because they activate the genetic mechanism for programmed cell death [apoptosis]. Finally, the cell disintegrates. In-

hibitory interneurons are particularly sensitive to excitotoxicity, which tonically express the activity of nociceptive central neurons. Therefore, after such a process, the input region of the strong nociceptive input is devoid of inhibitory interneurons, and the nociceptive neurons in that area are chronically disinhibited and hyperactive. This mechanism may be of importance for patients who develop fibromyalgia pain after a whiplash injury (27).

When such structural changes in the central nervous system have occurred, treatment of pain cannot be expected to have immediate success because the alterations in spinal circuitry take time to normalize, if they normalize at all.

THE POTENTIAL ROLE OF GLIAL CELLS IN CENTRAL SENSITIZATION INDUCED BY A PAINFUL MUSCLE LESION

In recent years, it has become apparent that both neuron-glia and glia-neuron signalling is likely to occur. Concerning lesion-induced neuroplastic changes, glial cells are uniquely positioned to alter neuronal responsiveness and synaptic function (28). Astrocytes are involved in the formation of synapses and modulation of synaptic transmission (29,30). Since microglia and astrocytes produce neuroactive substances that are involved in nociception (31,32), it is reasonable to assume that glial cells play a role in nociceptive processing. Actually, these cells appear to be involved in central sensitization (30) and in the development of allodynia and hyperalgesia (33). Interestingly, astrocytes also produce the fibroblast growth factor 2 [FGF-2], especially under pathophysiological conditions (34), which is extremely effective in *depressing* all kinds of neuronal activity (35). Thus, it seems that there is a massive excitatory-inhibitory influence between astroglial and neuronal cells under physiological and pathophysiological conditions.

Preliminary data obtained in our laboratory show that in fact astrocytes [the most frequent glial cells in the spinal cord] are strongly influenced by a painful lesion of a peripheral muscle. The aim of the study was to find out if a chronic experimental myositis is associated with alterations of astrocytic morphology, and changes in the synthesis of glial fibrillary acidic protein [GFAP] and FGF-2. Glial fibrillary acidic pro-

tein is an astrocyte-specific cytoskeletal protein that is necessary for the formation of stable astrocytic processes; it has been shown to react in a sensitive way to pathophysiological situations (31,33,36). Fibroblast growth factor 2 synthesized by astrocytes can influence the activity of neurons, since one member of the FGF-receptor family [FGFR-1] is located preferentially on neurons The two latter factors were determined with immunohistochemical methods and quantitatively evaluated.

After 12 days of an experimental myositis of the GS muscle, the amount of GFAP in the dorsal horn was significantly increased. The shape factor–which describes how close the outline of a structure is to an exact circle–likewise exhibited a significant increase. Apparently, under the influence of the peripheral myositis the astrocyte morphology changed so that its outline became plumper.

As shown in Figure 5B, the number of FGF-2-positive nuclei increased significantly in the spinal dorsal horn and intermediate substance of myositis animals. Double staining for FGF-2-immunoreactivity [IR] and GFAP-IR

FIGURE 5. Myositis-induced changes in FGF-2 immunoreactivity [IR]. **A.** Double staining for FGF-2 and GFAP. Arrows indicate FGF-2-immunoreactive [ir, dark diaminobenzidine [DAB]-reaction] nuclei surrounded by fluorescent GFAP-IR. **B.** Number of spinal cells with FGF-2-ir nuclei [ipsilateral to the myositis, expressed as number of immunoreactive nuclei per tissue section. Open bars, animals with intact GS muscle; black bars, animals with inflamed muscle, duration of inflammation 12 d [*, P < 0.01; ***, P < 0.001]. Roman numerals underneath the bars indicate the laminae of the dorsal horn.

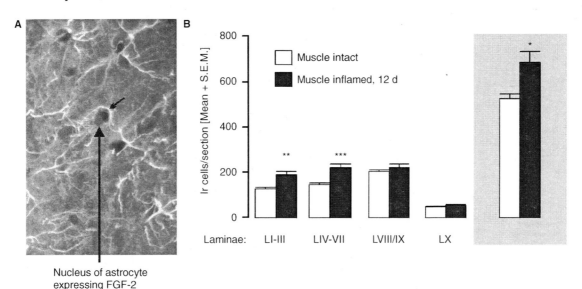

showed that all FGF-2-IR nuclei were located in astrocytes [Figure 5A].

The data show that spinal astrocytes react with GFAP hypertrophy and morphological changes to an inflammation in a peripheral muscle. The observed reorientation of the astrocytic processes might be of importance for changes in nociceptive transmission during chronic pain. Hadley and Ghoshgarian (37) postulated changes in neuronal excitability following retraction of astrocyte processes. There are also data showing that acute peripheral inflammation causes glial activation that correlates with pain behavior in the rat (33).

As to the neuronal effects of the increased FGF-2 synthesis in astrocytes, data of our group showed that in addition to the well-known neurotrophic actions, FGF-2 directly influenced the impulse activity of dorsal horn neurons (35). As the influence of FGF-2 on neurons consisted of a strong inhibition of electrical activity, and as FGF-2 expression is increased under painful pathophysiological conditions, FGF-2 may constitute a factor that counteracts the transition from acute to chronic pain.

REFERENCES

1. Wall PD, Woolf CJ: Muscle but not cutaneous C-afferent input produces prolonged increases in the excitability of the flexion reflex in the rat. J Physiol 356: 443-458, 1984.

2. Hoheisel U, Koch K, Mense S: Functional reorganization in the rat dorsal horn during an experimental myositis. Pain 59:111-118, 1994.

3. Woolf CJ, Salter MW: Neuronal plasticity: Increasing the gain in pain. Science 288:1765-1768, 2000.

4. Baranauskas G, Nistri A: Sensitization of pain pathways in the spinal cord: Cellular mechanisms. Prog Neurobiol 54:349-365, 1998.

5. Hoheisel U, Sander B, Mense S: Myositis-induced functional reorganization of the rat dorsal horn: Effects of spinal superfusion with antagonists to neurokinin and glutamate receptors. Pain 69:219-230, 1997.

6. Hoheisel U, Sander B, Mense S: Blockade of nitric oxide synthase differentially influences background activity and electrical excitability in rat dorsal horn neurons. Neurosci Lett 188:143-146, 1995.

7. De Vere R, Bradley WG: Polymyositis: its presentation, morbidity, and mortality. Brain 98:637-666, 1975.

8. Ansell BM: Management of polymyositis and dermatomyositis. Clin Rheum Dis 10. edited by BM Ansell. Saunders, London, pp. 205-213, 1984.

9. Knowles RG, Palacios M, Palmar RM, Moncada S: Formation of nitric oxide from L-arginine in the central nervous system: A transduction mechanism for stimulation of the soluble guanylate cyclase. Proc Natl Acad Sci USA 86:5159-5162, 1989.

10. Haley JE, Dickenson AH, Schachter M: Electrophysiological evidence for a role of nitric oxide in prolonged chemical nociception in the rat. Neuropharm 31:251-258, 1992.

11. Meller ST, Gebhart GF: Nitric oxide (NO) and nociceptive processing in the spinal cord. Pain 52:127-136, 1993.

12. Semos ML, Headley PM: The role of nitric oxide in spinal nociceptive reflexes in rats with neurogenic and non-neurogenic peripheral inflammation. Neuropharmacol 33:1487-1497, 1994.

13. Duarte ID, Ferreira SD: L-NAME causes antinociception by stimulation of the arginine-NO-cGMP pathway. Mediators Inflamm 9:25-30, 2000.

14. Tegeder I, Schmidtko A, Niederberger E, Ruth P, Geisslinger G: Dual effects of spinally delivered 8-bromo-cyclic guanosine monophosphate (8-bromo-cGMP) in formalin-induced nociception in rats. Neurosci Lett 332:146-150, 2002.

15. Pehl U, Schmid HA: Electrophysiological responses of neurons in the rat spinal cord to nitric oxide. Neurosci 77:563-573, 1997.

16. Manjarrez E, Rocha T, Rojas-Piloni G, Mendez I, Flores A: Nitric oxide modulates spontaneous cord dorsum potentials in the cat spinal cord. Neurosci Lett 309:5-8, 2001.

17. Hoheisel U, Unger T, Mense S: A block of spinal nitric oxide synthesis leads to increased background activity predominantly in nociceptive dorsal horn neurones in the rat. Pain 88:249-257, 2000.

18. Goldstein I, Lue TF, Padma-Nathan H, Rosen RC, Steers, WD, Wicker, PA: Oral sildenafil in the treatment of erectile dysfunction. New Engl J Med 338: 1397-1404, 1998.

19. Olsson AM, Speakman MJ, Dinsmore WW, Giuliano F, Gingell C, Maytom M, Smith MD, Osterley I: Sildenafil citrate (Viagra) is effective and well tolerated for treating erectile dysfunction of psychogenic or mixed aetiology. Int J Clin Pract 54:561-566, 2000.

20. Lim PH, Ng FC, Cheng CW, Wong MY, Chee CT, Moorthy P, Vasan SS: Clinical safety profile of sildenafil in Singaporean men with erectile dysfunction: Pre-marketing experience (ASSESS-I evaluation). J Int Med Res 30:137-143, 2002.

21. Milman HA, Arnold SB: Neurologic, psychological, and aggressive disturbances with sildenafil. Ann Pharmacotherapy 36:1129-1134, 2002.

22. Fields HL, Basbaum AI: Central nervous system mechanisms of pain modulation. In: Textbook of Pain, edited by Wall PD, Melzack R, Harcourt, London, pp. 309-329, 1999.

23. Duggan AW, Morton CR: Tonic descending inhibition and spinal nociceptive transmission. Prog Brain Res 77:193-211, 1989 (publisher's limited).

24. Sandkühler J: The organisation and function of endogenous antinociceptive systems. Prog Neurobiol 50:49-81, 1996.

25. Millan MJ: Descending control of pain. Prog Neurobiol 66:355-474, 2002.

26. Yezierski RP, Liu S, Ruenes GL, Kajander KJ, Brewer KL: Excitotoxic spinal cord injury: Behavioral and morphological characteristics of a central pain model. Pain 75:141-155, 1998.

27. Buskila D, Neumann L, Vaisberg G: Increased rates of fibromyalgia following cervical spinal injury: A controlled study of 161 cases of traumatic injury. Arthritis Rheum 40:446-452, 1997.

28. Anderson CM, Swanson RA: Astrocyte glutamate transport: Review of properties, regulation, and physiological functions. Glia 32:1-14, 2000.

29. Haydon PG: Glia: Listening and talking to synapse, Nature Rev. Neurosci 2:185-193, 2001.

30. Ma JY, Zhao ZQ: The involvement of glia in long-term plasticity in the spinal dorsal horn of the rat. Neuroreport, 13:1781-1784, 2003.

31. Watkins, L.R: Spinal cord glia: New players in pain. Pain 93:201-205, 2001.

32. Watkins LR, Maier SF: Glia: A novel drug discovery target for clinical pain. Nature Rev 2:973-985, 2003.

33. Sweitzer SM, Colburn RW, Rutkowski M, DeLeo JA: Acute peripheral inflammation induces moderate glial activation and spinal IL-1β expression that correlates with pain behavior in the rat. Brain Res 829:209-221, 1999.

34. Madiai F, Hussain SR, Goettl VM, Burry RW, Stephens RL Jr, Hackshaw KV: Upregulation of FGF-2 in reactive spinal cord astrocytes following unilateral lumbar spinal nerve ligation. Exp Brain Res 148:366-376, 2003.

35. Blüm T, Hoheisel U, Unger T, Mense S: Fibroblast growth factor-2 acutely influences the impulse activity of rat dorsal horn neurones. Neurosci Res 40:115-123, 2001.

36. McCann MJ, O'Callaghan JP, Martin PM, Bertram T, Streit WJ: Differential activation of microglia and astrocytes following trimethyl tin-induced neurodegeneration. Neurosci 72:273-281, 1996.

37. Hadley SD, Goshgarian HG: Altered immunoreactivity for glial fibrillary acidic protein in astrocytes within 1h after cervical spinal cord injury. Exp Neurol 146:380-387, 1997.

Therapy for Idiopathic Low Back Pain

H. Bliddal

SUMMARY. Objectives: To describe the importance of distinguishing between specific and non-specific therapies offered in low back pain [LBP].

Findings: In acute LBP, manual treatments or specific exercises may shorten the duration of the attack, while long-term effects of these interventions have not been proven. In the individual case, finding and treating a myofascial source of the pain may alter the course of the disease, while these cases apparently vary too much to be studied in regular controlled series. In chronic LBP, specific therapy should be avoided and replaced by active rather than passive therapies. The results of any of the therapies depend on the personality of the therapist and a large placebo effect is encountered.

Conclusions: The reassurance of the patient is a very important factor influencing the prognosis. The choice of therapy should take into account the plausibility, safety, cost-effectiveness, and feasibility of the intervention. *[Article copies available for a fee from The Haworth Document Delivery Service: 1-800-HAWORTH. E-mail address: <docdelivery@haworthpress.com> Website: <http://www. HaworthPress.com>* © 2004 by The Haworth Press, Inc. All rights reserved.]

KEYWORDS. Case history, clinical examination, diagnosis, specificity, intervention

INTRODUCTION

The obvious medical approach to any patient is to collect data by the case history, examine the area in question, based on these clinical findings supplement with laboratory or imaging analysis and then prescribe a treatment to cure the disease. Having done this, the therapist will give some good advice as to prevent recurrence of the disease and according to schedule the ex-patient will then carry on as a healthy subject in the background population and not bother the medical system anymore.

This train of events happens all the time in the medical profession and is often a source of fulfillment for the therapist, just like solving a riddle or getting the right answer in a complicated mathematical equation. Such happy outcome would be expected after diagnosing and treating pneumococcus pneumonia with penicillin.

Systematically, the medical diagnosis and treatments may be shown in a 2 × 2 table [Figure 1], indicating that diagnoses may be divided into specific and non-specific and, similarly, treatments into specific and non-specific. This is a very simplistic breakdown of much more complicated matters; however, the classification may be used to highlight some of our troubles in the therapy of low-back pain [LBP]. In general medicine, examples may be found in the four subclasses.

While in the musculoskeletal system specific Class A cases are few and far between, the recollection of spectacular successes is nevertheless typical to almost any profession dealing with these cases. There are some examples that

H. Bliddal, MD, is Professor, Parker Institute, Frederiksberg Hospital, Ndr Fasanvej 57, Denmark DK-2000 [E-mail: hb@fh.hosp.dk].

[Haworth co-indexing entry note]: "Therapy for Idiopathic Low Back Pain." Bliddal, H. Co-published simultaneously in *Journal of Musculoskeletal Pain* [The Haworth Medical Press, an imprint of The Haworth Press, Inc.] Vol. 12, No. 3/4, 2004, pp. 111-119; and: *Soft Tissue Pain Syndromes: Clinical Diagnosis and Pathogenesis* [ed: Dieter E. Pongratz, Siegfried Mense, and Michael Spaeth] The Haworth Medical Press, an imprint of The Haworth Press, Inc., 2004, pp. 111-119. Single or multiple copies of this article are available for a fee from The Haworth Document Delivery Service [1-800-HAWORTH, 9:00 a.m. - 5:00 p.m. [EST]. E-mail address: docdelivery@haworthpress.com].

FIGURE 1. A diagram with four general possibilities of combinations of diagnosis and therapy. The effectiveness of a remedy or treatment will depend on the specificity of both dimensions. Despite this uncertainty, in the single patient the outcome may be determined by luck.

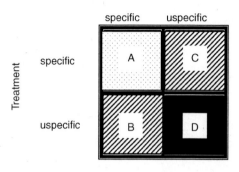

Class A: This will imply a certain diagnosis given a specific treatment directed against this known abnormality. An example would be an antibiotic treatment against a microorganism after proper resistance testing.

Class B: A certain diagnosis has been given to a case, which cannot be offered a specific therapy, while treated with unspecific means. Example: Diuretics and morphine given to a patient with pulmonary congestion [cardiac failure].

Class C: The diagnosis is uncertain, however, a specific therapy is given directed against a specific structure or biochemical entity. Example: Antipyretics given to the patient with high fever.

Class D: Neither specific diagnosis, nor specific therapy is possible. Example: Pain killers for headache.

approach this ideal: it could be the diagnosis—both clinical and by imaging—of localized pain in a finger or hand due to an acute tenosynovitis. This could be cured by local injection of glucocorticoids and with proper changes of loading of the tendon a recurrence might be avoided.

It may be postulated that a Class A situation never occurs in the low-back. A seemingly clear-cut situation as acute disc herniation results in a physical lesion from the pressure and is additionally complicated by a varying degree of inflammation of the perineurium of the nerve-root along with myofascial syndromes in the adjacent soft tissues. The management of LBP will have to take the psychological aspects of pain therapy into account. Any given case of LBP will be presented by a patient giving his or her version of the pain through a filter of language, culture, and acquired pain behavior. On the receptive side, the therapist has a similar filter to translate the signals and transform this into a meaningful intervention. A lot of cultural

and social factors determine how reactions are to the therapeutic efforts.

To make everything even more complicated the final evaluation of the effectiveness of the therapy must come through yet another filtration process with personal, social, and economic sideline to be accounted for. The process line may be illustrated as shown in Figure 2.

In each step of this process from lesion to measurement of outcome, a variation will be introduced. Each of the confounders of this kind would be expected to add bias and provided they are additive, a net result of considerable variation is expected. With a longer duration of the LBP, these confounders have more time to act, the reaction in the central nervous system may spread and in the chronic situation the importance of the original lesion may very well be lost.

MANY TYPES OF THERAPY

Therapy of LBP may be divided into nonspecific measures to relieve the pain and more specific interventions against the lesion causing the pain. The specific therapeutic ideas would have the best chances in the acute phases of LBP, when chronicity of the pain sensations has not yet been established.

To exemplify, in the acute phase the patient with a herniated disc should be relieved by a

FIGURE 2. Possible confounders in the process of low back pain from lesion to outcome.

Lesion	Patient modulation
	Society factors
	Therapist empathy
	Therapeutic possibility
Diagnosis	Therapist education
	Patient reaction to label
	Socioeconomic
Treatment	Therapist expectations
	Patient reaction to physical contact
	Politeness
	Socioeconomic
Outcome	Measurement instruments

medication against both pain and the local inflammatory reaction, preferably a non-steroidal anti-inflammatory drug. Also, a more specific intervention might be needed, ultimately an operation.

It must, however, be realized that most cases of acute LBP will be cured by nature. All therapeutic efforts in the acute phases of LBP can be regarded as accelerators of the natural cure. An example of this axiomatic course has been given in the study of Mathews et al. (1), showing beautifully the spontaneous cure in the reference group ending with a frequency of persistent pain at exactly the same level as the intervention. The statistical possibility of success with a given therapy in these circumstances is at least in the same order as the rate of spontaneous cure, provided the treatment is not harmful by itself.

These factors combined with a general tendency of "doctor-shopping" for LBP that does not remit within a short while (2) may be one explanation for the numerous therapies offered for LBP. Accordingly, no single entity has been able to demonstrate its advantage over the other.

REGIONAL PAIN DISORDERS IN LOW BACK PAIN

The case history including the localization of the pain and the extension into the leg are the most important background information, while imaging and neurological tests add little diagnostic value even in the case of a disc herniation (3).

In the main part of cases, a sound diagnostic effort leads to the exclusion of a number of well known diseases and limits the diagnostic possibilities within the frames of a regional pain disorder. An extension of the LBP into the lower extremity will reduce the possible diagnoses [Table 1].

Discogenic pain cannot by extension only be distinguished from the referred pain from muscles (4). Syndromes of pain referral from the muscles are important to recognize not to have the treatment misguided by a faulty diagnosis. There are, however, severe problems of designation and terminology, which may be reduced by training the therapists. It is quite obvious that

further diagnosis of such conditions, "syndromes," are dependent on the collaboration of the patient and the skill and experience of the therapist (5).

The diagnosis of most of the myofascial syndromes is more difficult in the sense that it cannot be proven. Few of these syndromes are present in a sufficient number for research purposes, which makes the experience with therapy less predictable than if the treatment plan were based on studies with larger cohorts of patients. The existence of the syndromes is substantiated by the reports of rather favorable reproducibility of the clinical examination, in all cases performed by highly specialized examiners (6,7).

BED REST

Two quite opposite principles in the reaction to pain including musculoskeletal problems are encountered in both the layman and the professional attitudes: either we try to cure by rest or we try to motion/train/exercise ["desperate ill need desperate remedies"]. For long periods of our recent history, these two opposite tendencies have alternated to set the fashion.

As for LBP, the natural thing in the acute phase is to lie down. This helps immediately on the pain and has been proven effective in some studies of acute LBP (8). The bed rest should not be prolonged as this will apparently only have an effect on the days lost from work (9). Due to the inactivity bed rest is potentially harmful and should be avoided or limited to a very short duration, when possible (10,11).

EXTENSION EXERCISES

It is debated, which structure is the most common source of the pain, and the discus seems to be a very relevant candidate (12). The McKenzie-system for diagnosis and treatment of LBP has as mainstay the notion of the discus as primary origin of the pain and gives a thorough subdivision into several major categories of discus disease (13). By far the most common discus pathology is the disc protrusion and this may be relieved by extension exercises in a substantial number of patients (14).

TABLE 1. Possible Reasons for Complaints of Low Back Pain [LBP].

Low back pain without irradiation	LBP irradiation to the thigh	LBP irradiation below the knee
Discus degeneration	Discus degeneration	Discus herniation
Discus herniation	Discus herniation	Kissing spine
Spondylosis	Kissing spine	Spinal stenosis
Spondylarthrosis	Spinal stenosis	Facet syndrome
Kissing spine	Facet syndrome	Myofascial pain syndromes
Arcolysis/spondylolisthesis	Myofascial pain syndromes	Fibromyalgia syndrome
Scheuermann	Fibromyalgia syndrome	
Spinal stenosis		
Fracture [Osteoporosis]		
Facet syndrome		
Ligament-pain		
Sacroiliac dysfunction		
Myelomatosis		
Neoplasia		
Spondylitis		
Spondylarthritis		
Muscle pain NB including psoas		
Renal diseases		
Abdominal tumours		
Obstipation		
Pelvic disorders		
Menstruation pain		
Endometriosis		
Medical diseases [Thyroid, Hypocalcemia]		
Herpes zoster		
Myofascial pain syndromes		
Fibromyalgia syndrome		

The list is not meant to be all-encompassing, while demonstrating the large number of differential diagnoses, when not associated with irradiation to the lower extremity.

Indirectly, the McKenzie approach presumes that discus material may be moved from the back of the arch and pushed forward towards less painful and more innocuous positions of a troubled disc. There is circumstantial evidence for the benefits of extension of the back in this respect although the effect varies much between individuals (15,16).

The system is easily understandable for both therapists and patients, which is of great importance for the chances of therapy (17,18). The more rigorous extension exercises may cause some local irritation of the low-back and in our experience passive extensions are just as effec-tive [Rasmussen et al., unpublished]. Such ma-neuvers may be implemented in the everyday life of a typical desk-worker.

The passive extension exercises may be advocated as a sort of screening test in combination with therapy. Patients are asked to return after 14 days with a diary stating how many times these exercises have been performed during the day. Whether the effect of this is the extension maneuver by itself or the confidence on the part of the patient that this is the right treatment cannot be distinguished. As long as health is the outcome, the society and patients fare well with either possibility (19).

MANIPULATION

Manipulation is very popular in all phases of LBP. Many therapists have the manipulative instrument in their armamentarium and the patients are happy with a treatment that gives a quick response, which is even felt as a "whack." The mechanism of the instant relief seems to be a reflex inhibition of the muscles, e.g., the multifidus muscle, in combination with a modulation of the neuromuscular control (20). It is quite possible that this can be of value in the acute phases of LBP (21) and in skilled settings, subgroups eligible for this therapy may be determined with the strongest association to success being that of short duration of symptoms (22). Manipulation may by some be regarded as a highly specific intervention; however, this is not an exception from the general rule in LBP that psychological factors play a very important role in the outcome (23). In spite of some previous positive results with manipulation as therapy in chronic LBP (24), this is not advocated in most recent guidelines for therapy of chronic LBP (25). The adverse reactions to manipulation should be taken into account (26), even if the therapy may appear cost-effective (27).

PREVENTION OF RECURRENCE

Even after recovery, the seemingly healthy person will statistically be in between attacks rather than cured of disease (28,29). Presumably, permanent lesions in one or more structures mark most LBP patients, e.g., a degenerated disc. The prevalence of radiological disc degeneration is very high in the population and in younger people with LBP degenerative signs on magnetic resonance imaging are definitely associated with recurrent back pain (30). In addition, a diseased neuromuscular function of the segment, e.g., the multifidus muscle may need attention after recovery of the attack of acute LBP (31).

Almost any patient with chronic LBP will experience short lasting exacerbations of the pain, which may be difficult to tell from cases of 'pure' acute LBP. The lack of specific diagnosis and means of monitoring therapy are part of the background for a large number of different therapeutic measures.

In the main part of cases, a sound diagnostic effort leads to the exclusion of a number of well known diseases and leaves the patient and therapist with an ill defined regional disorder characterized by chronic pain.

Apparently, a well functioning tertiary prevention program will reduce the recurrence rate significantly (32). The patient's view upon the therapy is of great importance (33) and the mere confidence in a thorough instruction about the disease may alter the course considerably (19, 34,35). On the other hand, the confidence in therapy may by itself lead to a longer patient-relationship with a certain dependence on the therapy, by itself a sort of chronicity, as demonstrated in the case of long-term chiropractic therapy (18).

Comparisons between various interventions have not been convincing as to the effect of the single therapy. Intensive back exercises have been advocated by several groups, often in combination with large programs of functional restoration (36,37). Any late effect of such costly therapy has not been shown (38,39).

By consequence, therapy against LBP must include both psychological and somatic factors and thoroughness in examination and instruction has been shown *per se* to have a major impact on prognosis and preferably the patient should be dealt with in this way early in the course of the disease. Following the same line of thought, most guidelines of therapy against non-acute LBP advocate a generalized approach with emphasis on exercises to help the patient break out of a vicious circle of pain-promoting behavior with elements of pain, lack of physical activity, muscle weakness, and–in the end–social incompetence.

MEDICATION FOR LOW BACK PAIN

In major series, medication may relieve the patient of some of the troubles from the LBP (40), and it seems established that non-steroidal anti-inflammatory agents are slightly more efficient than the other analgesics (41). This is quite in line with the notion of inflammatory agents being liberated in the discus (42). In some contrast with this idea, potent anti-inflammatory treatment with local steroid therapy has not been proven efficacious when injected directly into the disc (43). A short-term effect may also be found with epidural steroid injections (44), which may be accompanied by adverse events limiting their applicability (45). In conclusion, medication for LBP may make coping with pain possible; however, this does not affect the final outcome.

SURGERY FOR LOW BACK PAIN

The necessity of operations in cases with severe neurological complications, e.g., an acute cauda equina syndrome, is not questioned. In all other cases of LBP a similar unanimous attitude has not been reached. The pro et contras concerning instrumentation are not settled and there are large methodological difficulties in proving the arguments. The cases subjected to these operations are characterized by problems of exact pain diagnosis including the psychological factors of chronic pain, which will confound the issue. As a matter of course, a double blind study is not possible and the primary outcome measures are mainly subjective patient reports.

The experience is only casuistic with most of the more recently developed operative treatments employing instrumentation of the spine. Regarding fusion for chronic, unspecific LBP, two randomized controlled studies have reached opposite conclusions; in a Swedish multicenter study, the group of patients treated with spine fusion had better pain relief than did controls with physical therapy (46), while a study in Norway using only one center of physical therapy showed equal results of fusion and cognitive intervention and exercises (47). It may once again be suspected that well determined therapists may alter the outcome considerably and that in this case physiotherapy as comparator displays a large variation from site to site. This is quite understandable from the above-mentioned effect of patient assurance (19) and should be taken into account in the planning of future studies.

ALTERNATIVE THERAPY

While a large percentage of patients take one or several kinds of complementary alternative medications [CAM] (48), none of these remedies are well studied and the expert's opinion of CAM for LBP is very low (49). Referring to the considerations above of specificity of the treatments in LBP, the question of using CAM as part of the treatment cannot be answered in general, while this may in the individual situation be of some value.

WHICH THERAPY TO CHOOSE?

In many cases, taking off the more strenuous work and shuffling a bit around a few days seems to be a good piece of advice in case of acute LBP (50). In any case, it has been very difficult to demonstrate any major advantage of exercises, manipulations, or other of the often prescribed therapies (51). Indeed, there seems to be a very substantial amount of placebo-effect in the results (52). Thus, gifted therapists with convincing and exciting new therapies have a good chance of actually affecting the outcome for their patients. Examples of such are neuroreflexotherapy (53), combination of steroid injection with manipulation (54), and electromyographic biofeedback (55). With any intervention, there is a possibility of adverse effects. Acknowledging the benign nature of LBP, the interventions chosen should be without significant risks to the patients. This would be a prerequisite for accepting or rejecting therapies. On the other hand, the patients have a natural demand for something to be done. In some cases, the actual amount and number of interventions, rather than the single instrument seems to be determining the outcome (56). An indication of insatiable treatment demands in patients with chronic LBP was seen in the fact that a significant part of the participants in the intensive functional restoration programs took extra therapy (36).

The thoroughbred idea of convincing the patients of self-cure rather than actually providing therapy has been tested in the Swedish back-school as discussed (57). It seems that a basic requirement for the success of such intervention is an enigmatic person leading the program (35). In conclusion, as long as no specific lesion may be demonstrated in LBP, a program should be sought that fulfills the following demands:

- Plausible
- Active rather than passive
- Safe
- Cost-effective
- Feasible

The result of these considerations will by necessity lead to different approaches according to cultural, educational, and economical factors. There is not much guidance to be found in the individual patient/therapist situation in the National guidelines, which inevitably come to the conclusion that non-specific measures are the only "evidence-based" treatments (25). The mainstay of therapy will be a diagnosis sufficiently specific to rule out differential diagnoses and at the same time allowing the therapist to engage in a professionally well founded intervention.

REFERENCES

1. Mathews JA, Mills SB, Jenkins VM, Grimes SM, Morkel MJ, Mathews W, Scott CM, Sittampalam Y: Back pain and sciatica: Controlled trials of manipulation, traction, sclerosant and epidural injections. Br J Rheumatol 26(6):416-423, 1987.

2. Nickel R, Egle UT, Rompe J, Eysel P, Hoffmann SO: Somatization predicts the outcome of treatment in patients with low back pain. J Bone Joint Surg Br 84(2): 189-195, 2002.

3. Albeck MJ: A critical assessment of clinical diagnosis of disc herniation in patients with monoradicular sciatica. Acta Neurochir (Wien) 138(1):40-44, 1996.

4. Simons DG, Travell JG: Myofascial origins of low back pain. 1. Principles of diagnosis and treatment. Postgrad Med 73(2):66, 68-70, 73, 1983.

5. McCombe PF, Fairbank JC, Cockersole BC, Pynsent PB: 1989 Volvo Award in clinical sciences: Reproducibility of physical signs in low-back pain. Spine 14(9):908-918, 1989.

6. Hsieh CY, Hong CZ, Adams AH, Platt KJ, Danielson CD, Hoehler FK, Tobis JS: Interexaminer reliability of the palpation of trigger points in the trunk and lower limb muscles. Arch Phys Med Rehabil 81(3): 258-264, 2000.

7. Strender LE, Sjoblom A, Sundell K, Ludwig R, Taube A: Interexaminer reliability in physical examination of patients with low back pain. Spine 22(7):814-820, 1997.

8. Wiesel SW, Cuckler JM, Deluca F, Jones F, Zeide MS, Rothman RH: Acute low-back pain: An objective analysis of conservative therapy. Spine 5(4): 324-330, 1980.

9. Deyo RA, Diehl AK, Rosenthal M: How many days of bed rest for acute low back pain? A randomized clinical trial. N Engl J Med 315(17):1064-1070, 1986.

10. Allen C, Glasziou P, Del Mar C: Bed rest: A potentially harmful treatment needing more careful evaluation. Lancet 354(9186):1229-1233, 1999.

11. Hagen KB, Hilde G, Jamtvedt G, Winnem MF: The Cochrane review of advice to stay active as a single treatment for low back pain and sciatica. Spine 27(16): 1736-1741, 2002.

12. Schwarzer AC, Aprill CN, Derby R, Fortin J, Kine G, Bogduk N: The prevalence and clinical features of internal disc disruption in patients with chronic low back pain. Spine 20(17):1878-1883, 1995.

13. Donelson R: The McKenzie approach to evaluating and treating low back pain. Orthop Rev 19(8):681-686, 1990.

14. Donelson R, Aprill C, Medcalf R, Grant W: A prospective study of centralization of lumbar and referred pain. A predictor of symptomatic discs and annular competence. Spine 22(10):1115-1122, 1997.

15. Adams MA, May S, Freeman BJ, Morrison HP, Dolan P: Effects of backward bending on lumbar intervertebral discs: Relevance to physical therapy treatments for low back pain. Spine 25(4):431-437, 2000.

16. Edmondston SJ, Song S, Bricknell RV, Davies PA, Fersum K, Humphries P, Wickenden D. Singer KP: MRI evaluation of lumbar spine flexion and extension in asymptomatic individuals. Man Ther 5(3):158-164, 2000.

17. Burton AK, Waddell G, Tillotson KM, Summerton N: Information and advice to patients with back pain can have a positive effect: A randomized controlled trial of a novel educational booklet in primary care. Spine 24(23): 2484-2491, 1999.

18. Goldstein MS, Morgenstern H, Hurwitz EL, Yu F: The impact of treatment confidence on pain and related disability among patients with low-back pain: Results from the University of California, Los Angeles, low-back pain study. Spine J 2(6):391-399, 2002.

19. Indahl A, Haldorsen EH, Holm S, Reikeras O, Ursin H: Five-year follow-up study of a controlled clinical trial using light mobilization and an informative approach to low back pain. Spine 23(23):2625-2630, 1998.

20. Dishman JD, Burke J: Spinal reflex excitability changes after cervical and lumbar spinal manipulation: A comparative study. Spine J 3(3):204-212, 2003.

21. van Tulder MW, Cherkin DC, Berman B, Lao L, Koes BW: The effectiveness of acupuncture in the management of acute and chronic low back pain: A systematic review within the framework of the Cochrane Collaboration Back Review Group. Spine 24(11): 1113-1123, 1999.

22. Flynn T, Fritz J, Whitman J, Wainner R, Magel J, Rendeiro D et al.: A clinical prediction rule for classifying patients with low back pain who demonstrate short-term improvement with spinal manipulation. Spine 27(24):2835-2843, 2002.

23. Hoehler FK, Tobis JS: Psychological factors in the treatment of back pain by spinal manipulation. Br J Rheumatol 22(4):206-212, 1983.

24. Meade TW, Dyer S, Browne W, Frank AO: Randomized comparison of chiropractic and hospital outpatient management for low back pain: Results from extended follow up. BMJ 311(7001):349-351, 1995.

25. Koes BW, van Tulder MW, Ostelo R, Kim BA, Waddell G: Clinical guidelines for the management of low back pain in primary care: An international comparison. Spine 26(22):2504-2513, 2001.

26. Haldeman S, Rubinstein SM: Cauda equina syndrome in patients undergoing manipulation of the lumbar spine. Spine 17(12):1469-1473, 1992.

27. Carey TS, Garrett J, Jackman A, McLaughlin C, Fryer J, Smucker DR: The outcomes and costs of care for acute low back pain among patients seen by primary care practitioners, chiropractors, and orthopedic surgeons: The North Carolina Back Pain Project. N Engl J Med 333(14):913-917, 1995.

28. Von Korff M, Saunders K: The course of back pain in primary care. Spine 21(24):2833-2837, 1996.

29. Wasiak R, Pransky G, Verma S, Webster B: Recurrence of low back pain: Definition-sensitivity analysis using administrative data. Spine 28(19):2283-2291, 2003.

30. Salminen JJ, Erkintalo MO, Pentti J, Oksanen A, Kormano MJ: Recurrent low back pain and early disc degeneration in the young. Spine 24(13):1316-1321, 1999.

31. Hides JA, Richardson CA, Jull GA: Multifidus muscle recovery is not automatic after resolution of acute, first-episode low back pain. Spine 21(23):2763-2769, 1996.

32. Garcy P, Mayer T, Gatchel RJ: Recurrent or new injury outcomes after return to work in chronic disabling spinal disorders: Tertiary prevention efficacy of functional restoration treatment. Spine 21(8):952-959, 1996.

33. Owens DK: Spine update: Patient preferences and the development of practice guidelines. Spine 23(9): 1073-1079, 1998.

34. Fordyce WE, Brockway JA, Bergman JA, Spengler D: Acute back pain: A control-group comparison of behavioral vs traditional management methods. J Behav Med 9(2):127-140, 1986.

35. Indahl A, Velund L, Reikeraas O: Good prognosis for low back pain when left untampered: A randomized clinical trial. Spine 20(4):473-477, 1995.

36. Mayer TG, Gatchel RJ, Mayer H, Kishino ND, Keeley J, Mooney V: A prospective two-year study of functional restoration in industrial low back injury: An objective assessment procedure. JAMA 258(13):1763-1767, 1987.

37. Manniche C, Asmussen K, Lauritsen B, Vinterberg H, Karbo H, Abildstrup S, Fischer-Nielsen K. Krebs R. Ibsen K: Intensive dynamic back exercises with or without hyperextension in chronic back pain after surgery for lumbar disc protrusion: A clinical trial. Spine 18(5): 560-567, 1993.

38. Bendix T, Bendix A, Labriola M, Haestrup C, Ebbehoj N: Functional restoration versus outpatient physical training in chronic low back pain: A randomized comparative study. Spine 25(19):2494-2500, 2000.

39. van Tulder MW, Malmivaara A, Esmail R, Koes BW: Exercise therapy for low back pain. Cochrane Database Syst Rev (2):CD000335, 2000.

40. Cherkin DC, Wheeler KJ, Barlow W, Deyo RA: Medication use for low back pain in primary care. Spine 23(5):607-614, 1998.

41. van Tulder MW, Scholten RJ, Koes BW, Deyo RA: Nonsteroidal anti-inflammatory drugs for low back pain: A systematic review within the framework of the Cochrane Collaboration Back Review Group. Spine 25(19):2501-2513, 2000.

42. Burke JG, Watson RW, McCormack D, Dowling FE, Walsh MG, Fitzpatrick JM: Intervertebral discs which cause low back pain secrete high levels of proinflammatory mediators. J Bone Joint Surg Br 84(2): 196-201, 2002.

43. Khot A, Bowditch M, Powell J, Sharp D: The use of intradiscal steroid therapy for lumbar spinal discogenic pain: A randomized controlled trial. Spine 29(8): 833-836, 2004.

44. Koes BW, Scholten RJ, Mens JM, Bouter LM: Efficacy of epidural steroid injections for low-back pain and sciatica: A systematic review of randomized clinical trials. Pain 63(3):279-288, 1995.

45. Young WF: Transient blindness after lumbar epidural steroid injection: A case report and literature review. Spine 27(21):E476-E477, 2002.

46. Fritzell P, Hagg O, Wessberg P, Nordwall A: 2001 Volvo Award Winner in Clinical Studies: Lumbar fusion versus nonsurgical treatment for chronic low back pain: A multicenter randomized controlled trial from the Swedish Lumbar Spine Study Group. Spine 26(23):2521-2532, 2001.

47. Ivar BJ, Sorensen R, Friis A, Nygaard O, Indahl A, Keller A, Ingebrigtsen T. Eriksen HR. Holm I. Koller AK. Riise R. Reikeras O: Randomized clinical trial of lumbar instrumented fusion and cognitive intervention and exercises in patients with chronic low back pain and disc degeneration. Spine 28(17):1913-1921, 2003.

48. Palinkas LA, Kabongo ML: The use of complementary and alternative medicine by primary care patients: A SURF*NET study. J Fam Pract 49(12):1121-1130, 2000.

49. Ernst E, Pittler MH: Experts' opinions on complementary/alternative therapies for low back pain. J Manipulative Physiol Ther 22(2):87-90, 1999.

50. Malmivaara A, Hakkinen U, Aro T, Heinrichs ML, Koskenniemi L, Kuosma E, Lappi S, Paloheimo R, Servo C, Vaaranen V: The treatment of acute low back pain–Bed rest, exercises, or ordinary activity? N Engl J Med 332(6):351-355, 1995.

51. Cherkin DC, Deyo RA, Battie M, Street J, Barlow W: A comparison of physical therapy, chiropractic ma-

nipulation, and provision of an educational booklet for the treatment of patients with low back pain. N Engl J Med 339(15):1021-1029, 1998.

52. Koes BW, Bouter LM, Knipshild PG, Van Mameren H, Essers A, Houben JP, Verstegen GM. Hofhuizen DM: The effectiveness of manual therapy, physiotherapy and continued treatment by the general practitioner for chronic nonspecific back and neck complaints: Design of a randomized clinical trial. J Manipulative Physiol Ther 14(9):498-502, 1991.

53. Kovacs FM, Abraira V, Pozo F, Kleinbaum DG, Beltran J, Mateo I, Perez de Ayala C. Pena A. Zea A. Gonzalez-Lanza M. Morillas L: Local and remote sustained trigger point therapy for exacerbations of chronic low back pain: A randomized, double-blind, controlled, multicenter trial. Spine 22(7):786-797, 1997.

54. Blomberg S, Hallin G, Grann K, Berg E, Sennerby U: Manual therapy with steroid injections–A new approach to treatment of low back pain: A controlled multicenter trial with an evaluation by orthopedic surgeons. Spine 19(5):569-577, 1994.

55. Hasenbring M, Ulrich HW, Hartmann M, Soyka D: The efficacy of a risk factor-based cognitive behavioral intervention and electromyographic biofeedback in patients with acute sciatic pain: An attempt to prevent chronicity. Spine 24(23):2525-2535, 1999.

56. Coxhead CE, Inskip H, Meade TW, North WR, Troup JD: Multicentre trial of physiotherapy in the management of sciatic symptoms. Lancet 1(8229):1065-1068, 1981.

57. Hall H, Hadler NM: Controversy: Low back school: Education or exercise? Spine 20(9):1097-1098, 1995.

INAUGURAL INCOMING PRESIDENT'S ADDRESS

Scientific Aspects and Clinical Signs of Muscle Pain

Dieter E. Pongratz
Matthias Vorgerd
Benedikt G. H. Schoser

SUMMARY. Objectives: The clinically most important painful muscle disorders are inflammatory and metabolic myopathies. In the three major groups of autoimmune inflammatory myopathies, dermatomyositis, polymyositis, and sporadic inclusion body myositis, muscle pain is most frequent in dermatomyositis and almost absent in sporadic inclusion body myositis.

Findings: The myopathological feature of dermatomyositis is polymyositis of the perifascicular type with pronounced inflammatory reaction of small blood vessels with C5B9 complement deposits and tubuloreticular inclusions as seen by electron microscopy. The last mentioned structures are induced by cytokines. Small free nerve endings are always connected to small blood vessels. In dermatomyositis one can show very clearly that substance P and calcitonine gene related peptide are elevated as signs of an increased nociceptive input. In polymyositis and especially inclusion body myositis there is no such muscular pathology and as far as examined no elevation of substance P and calcitonine gene related peptide in free nerve endings.

Many forms of metabolic myopathies, especially glycol[geno]lytic defects, are characterized by symptoms of exercise intolerance [early muscle fatigue, painful contractures with exercise, muscle cramps, myoglobinuria]. The investigation of muscle energy metabolism can be performed non-invasively by phosphorus magnetic resonance spectroscopy. The final diagnosis of the different forms depends on careful morphological and especially enzymatic studies. Pain after exercise is not well understood. Depletion of high-energy phosphates, like phosphocreatine and adenosine triphosphate during exercise, may contribute to the pathogenesis.

In the much more frequent local myofascial pain syndrome, caused by trigger points located

Dieter E. Pongratz, Prof. Dr. med., and Benedikt G. H. Schoser, Prov.-Doz. Dr. med., are affiliated with the Friedrich-Baur-Institute, Ludwig-Maximilians University, Munich, Germany.

Matthias Vorgerd, Prov.-Doz. Dr. med., is affiliated with the Department of Neurology, Ruhr-University of Bochum, Germany.

Address correspondence to: Dieter E. Pongratz, Prof. Dr. med., Friedrich-Baur-Institute, Ludwig-Maximilians University, Ziemssenstr. 1a, 80336 Munich, Germany [E-mail: dieter.pongratz@med.uni-muenchen.de].

The authors would like to thank Siegfried Mense, Heidelberg, Germany and Joseph Müller-Höcker, Munich, Germany for ongoing cooperation in this field.

[Haworth co-indexing entry note]: "Scientific Aspects and Clinical Signs of Muscle Pain." Pongratz, Dieter E., Matthias Vorgerd, and Benedikt G. H. Schoser. Co-published simultaneously in *Journal of Musculoskeletal Pain* [The Haworth Medical Press, an imprint of The Haworth Press, Inc.] Vol. 12, No. 3/4, 2004, pp. 121-128; and: *Soft Tissue Pain Syndromes: Clinical Diagnosis and Pathogenesis* [ed: Dieter E. Pongratz, Siegfried Mense, and Michael Spaeth] The Haworth Medical Press, an imprint of The Haworth Press, Inc., 2004, pp. 121-128. Single or multiple copies of this article are available for a fee from The Haworth Document Delivery Service [1-800-HAWORTH, 9:00 a.m. - 5:00 p.m. [EST]. E-mail address: docdelivery@haworthpress.com].

within the substance of human skeleton muscles, alteration is really difficult. In our understanding, so called contraction discs are the most frequent findings. Often, but not always, these contraction discs are located in a neuromuscular end plate region. Further human studies are ongoing.

Conclusions: We conclude that the morphopathogenetic background of muscle pain is still widely unclear. Free nerve endings, substance P and adenosine triphosphate and acidosis seems to be the major player in distinct neuromuscular disorders. *[Article copies available for a fee from The Haworth Document Delivery Service: 1-800-HAWORTH. E-mail address: <docdelivery@haworthpress. com> Website: <http://www.HaworthPress.com> © 2004 by The Haworth Press, Inc. All rights reserved.]*

KEYWORDS. Muscle pain, dermatomyositis, polymyositis, inclusion body myositis, metabolic myopathies, myofascial pain syndrome

INTRODUCTION

The clinically most important painful muscle disorders are acquired immunogenic inflammatory and inherited metabolic myopathies. There are three major groups of autoimmune inflammatory myopathies

- dermatomyositis,
- polymyositis, and
- sporadic inclusion body myositis.

Myalgia is most frequent in dermatomyositis and nearly absent in sporadic inclusion body myositis.

Dermatomyositis from a clinical point of view is mostly an acute disease. The age of onset varies from childhood to the elderly. There is an acute weakness of the proximal skeletal muscles combined with diffuse muscle pain. Muscle wasting is not prominent. Additional features are rash and calcinosis. The morphological feature of dermatomyositis is polymyositis of the perifascicular type caused by affections of the small intramuscular blood vessels with endothelial proliferation and tubulovesicular inclusions seen by electron microscopy (1-5). These structures are induced by cytokines. Perifascicular damage and atrophy are typical for dermatomyositis. Immunohistological methods reveal the cellular infiltrates consisting of B-lymphocytes and some CD4-positive lymphocytes [Figure 1A + B]. Additionally C5b9-complement deposits within small blood vessels and capillaries are very characteristic [Figure 1C]. In cooperation with S. Mense, Heidelberg, Germany, we could show very clearly that small nerve endings are always connected to small blood vessels [Figure 1D]. These nerve endings contain elevated substance P [Figure 1E] and calcitonine gene related peptide [Figure 1 F] as signs of an increased nociceptive input.

Idiopathic polymyositis is a disease occurring especially in adults. Its evolution in time is subacute or chronic. Muscle weakness and atrophy of the proximal muscles of the extremities are the most prominent features. Pain is not frequent and never prominent. Cutaneous lesions cannot be found.

The morphological picture is a diffuse polymyositis, especially with CD8-positive lymphocytes [Figure 2A + B]. Very characteristic is invasion of non-necrotic muscle fibers [Figure 2C]. There is no vascular pathology (1-5). As far as examined, an elevation of substance P and calcitonine gene related peptide in free nerve endings could not be detected.

Sporadic inclusion body myositis is the most chronic form of immunogenic inflammatory myopathies. It progresses slowly and is a disease of the elderly, affecting much more men than women. An asymmetric involvement of proximal and distal muscles of the extremities is typical. Atrophies are prominent. Myalgias never occur (1-4,6).

The morphological picture is characterized by rimmed vacuoles with eosinophilics cytoplasmic inclusions [Figure 2D]. At electron microscopy, the vacuoles correspond to autophagic vacuoles. Filamentous inclusions in the cytoplasm and nuclei are pathognomonic [Figure 2E]. Additionally there is a chronic diffuse polymyositis with CD8-positive lymphocytes. There is no vascular pathology and no involvement of free nerve endings.

FIGURE 1. Dermatomyositis: **A.** Hematoxilin-eosin stain shows pronounced intra- and perifasciular infiltration and muscle atrophy. **B.** Anti-CD-4 positive leukocytes in dermatomyositis. **C.** Anti C5B9 Complement positive vessel [arrow]. **D.** Diagram of the relation between intramuscular vessels, free-nerve-endings and skeletal muscle. **E.** Anti-substance-P immunostaining [red] of intramuscular nerve branches. **F.** Anti-calcitonin-gene related protein [CGRP] immunostaining [red] of intramuscular nerve branches [blue].

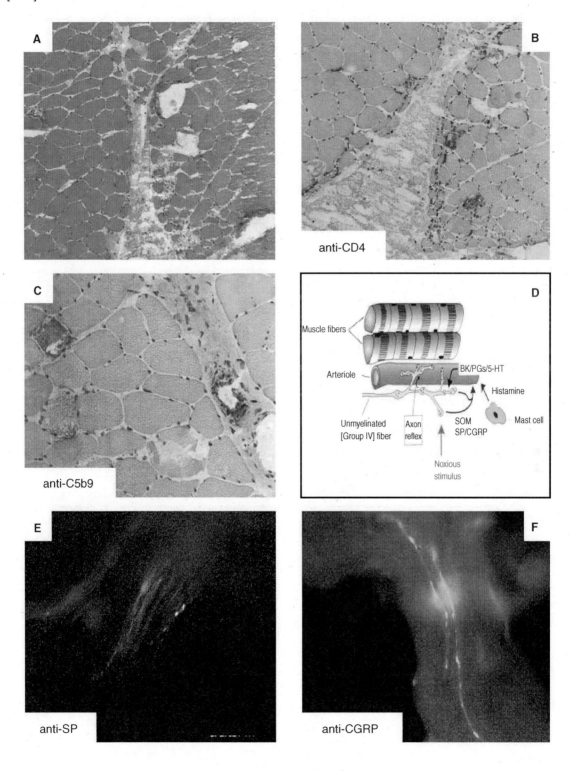

FIGURE 2. Polymyositis: **A.** Hematoxilin-eosin stain shows intrafascicular infiltration and myophagia with muscle necrosis. **B.** Anti-CD8 staining reveals massive intrafascicular infiltration of myofibers. **C.** Invasion of myofibers by CD-8 positive leukocytes. Inclusion body myositis: **D.** Hematoxilin-eosin stain shows typical rimmed vacuoles and myofiber degeneration with necrosis. **E.** Electron microscopy confirms inclusion body myositis by demonstrating intracellular and intranuclear fibrils.

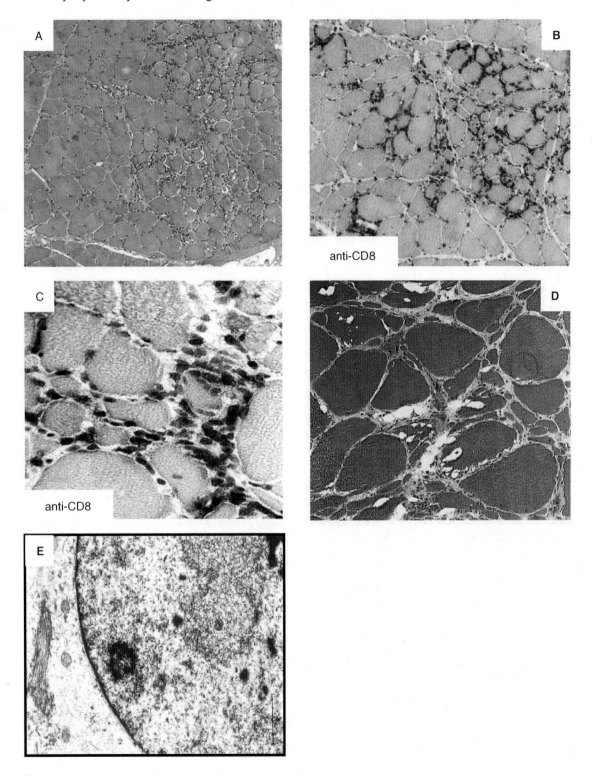

The group of inherited metabolic myopathies can be subdivided into glycogen storage diseases, lipid storage myopathies, mitochondrial myopathies and enzyme defects within the purine nucleotide cycle (1-4, 7-9).

The main clinical features are:

- progressive muscle weakness and atrophy [e.g., acid maltase deficiency],
- exercise intolerance with premature muscle fatigue, painful muscle contractures during exercise, muscle cramps and myoglobinuria [e.g., muscle phosphorylase deficiency], or
- recurrent rhabdomyolysis [e.g., carnitin-palmitoyl-transferase deficiency].

Phosphorus magnetic resonance spectroscopy [P-MRS] allows for direct, non-invasive investigation of muscle bioenergetics *in vivo*. Phosphorus magnetic resonance spectroscopy is conducted in high-field imaging systems and monitors energy metabolism during rest, exercise, and recovery from exercise. In human muscle, P-MRS spectra at rest contain five major peaks: three from the adenosine triphosphate, one from phosphocreatine, and one from inorganic phosphate [Figure 3A]. An additional peak from phosphomonoesters close to the inorganic phosphate peak is also often visible during exercise [Figure 3A].

Phosphorus magnetic resonance spectroscopy is a very useful diagnostic tool in patients with exercise intolerance and suspected metabolic myopathy. It is also helpful in monitoring therapeutic trials in metabolic myopathies, especially for novel therapies in mitochondrial and glycogen storage myopathies (7-9).

Skeletal muscle, with a primary defect in the cytosolic glycol[geno]lytic metabolism lack the ability to produce lactic acid during exercise and show an increase in the intracellular pH. This intracellular alkalinization is a very sensitive and specific spectroscopic finding in patients with a primary cytosolic glycol[geno]lytic enzyme defect [Figure 3B]. Moreover, P-MRS allows to distinguish glycolytic enzyme disorders such as Tarui's disease [phosphofructokinase deficiency, glycogenosis type VII] from glycogenolytic disorders by a huge accumulation of phosphomonoesters representing glucose-6-phosphate and fructose-6-phosphate (7-9).

Phosphorylase deficiency [McArdle disease, glycogenosis type V] is one of the most common muscle glycogenosis in adults. Histology reveals a vacuolar myopathy [Figure 3C] with negative histochemical phosphorylase staining [Figure 3D]. Phosphorus magnetic resonance spectroscopy in McArdle disease depicts a significant depletion of the high-energy phosphates adenosine triphosphate and phosphocreatine during aerobic and ischemic low-level exercise in addition to the increase in the intracellular pH [Figure 3E]. This reduction in the adenine nucleotide pool may lead to a failure of membrane excitation and impaired contractile mechanisms. Such an energy depletion may thus contribute to the typical clinical symptoms of painful muscle contractures, early fatigue, and muscle cramps beside other not yet identified metabolic alterations (1-4,7-9).

The most frequent metabolic myopathy is myoadenylate deaminase deficiency (1-4,10, 11). In this metabolic myopathy, a forearm exercise test cannot reveal an elevation of ammonia after exercise [Figure 3F + G]. The histochemistry shows a completely negative staining [Figure 3H]. Additional molecular biological studies are available (10,11). According to our experience some of these patients develop in the course of the disease a nearly typical picture of fibromyalgia that should be classified as secondary. A therapeutic intervention with D-Ribose can be successful.

In the much more frequent *local myofascial pain syndrome*, caused by trigger points, it is not easy to get human biopsy specimens (12-14). In the last months we had the opportunity to perform some biopsies with careful localization of trigger points by palpation, electromyography [end-plate potentials], and ultrasound [twitch response].

What we mostly have seen are contraction discs, often, but not always, located in an end-plate region [Figure 4A-C]. By electron microscopy one can show shortened Z-bands [Figure 4D], sometimes disturbance of the Z-line-structure [Figure 4E] together with some accumulation of structurally normal mitochondria in the subsarcolemmal region [Figure 4F]. Further human studies must be done in the future.

FIGURE 3. **A.** Phosphor-magnetic resonance spectroscopy [P-MRS] spectra of resting muscle [upper spectra] and after low-level exercise [lower spectra] from a healthy control person. Note the decline in PCr and the increase in Pi and PME with exercise, ATP remains constant. ATP = adenosine triphosphate; PCr = phosphocreatine; Pi = inorganic phosphate; PME = phosphomonoester; ppm = parts per million as a measure of the peak position in the spectrum. **B.** Intracellular pH during low-level aerobic [minutes 1 to 4 in the time scale] and ischaemic exercise [minutes 15 to 18 in the time scale] in 19 patients with phosphorylase deficiency [McArdle disease, glycogenosis type V] [filled circles] and in control persons [open circles]. In controls, the muscle pH becomes acidic, whereas in McArdle disease intracellular pH increases due to the inability to produce lactic acid. Values are mean ± SE. ** indicates no overlap of end exercise pH values in patients with the control range. **C.** McArdle disease histology: Vacuolar myopathy [left] with subsarcolemmal glycogen deposits [right]. **D.** Phosphorylase histochemistry demonstrates normal staining [left] compared to complete absence of phosphorylase activity in McArdle disease [right]. **E.** The level of phosphocreatine [PCr] during aerobic [minutes 1 to 4 in the time scale] and ischaemic exercise [minutes 15 to 18 in the time scale] in 19 patients with phosphorylase deficiency [filled circles] and in control persons [open circles]. Note the drastic decline of PCr in McArdle disease. Values are mean ± SE. * indicates significant lower levels of end exercise PCr values in patients. **F.** Fischer diagram of AMP-deaminase function. **G.** Lear-test demonstrates an impaired ammonia increase with normal lactate values in MAD patients. **H.** AMP-deaminase histochemistry. Compared to normal control [left] complete absence of AMP-desaminase activity in AMP-patient [right].

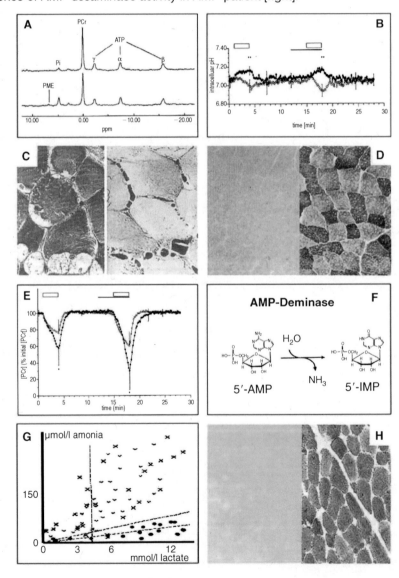

FIGURE 4. Endplate morphology and trigger point biopsy: **A.** Unspecific esterase staining demonstrates endplate region [blue]. **B-C.** Semithin section of a trigger point reveals contraction disk region. **D.** Electron microscopy shows shortened Z-bands and disturbance of the Z-line-structure, **E.** together with subsarcolemmal accumulation of structurally normal mitochondria **F.**

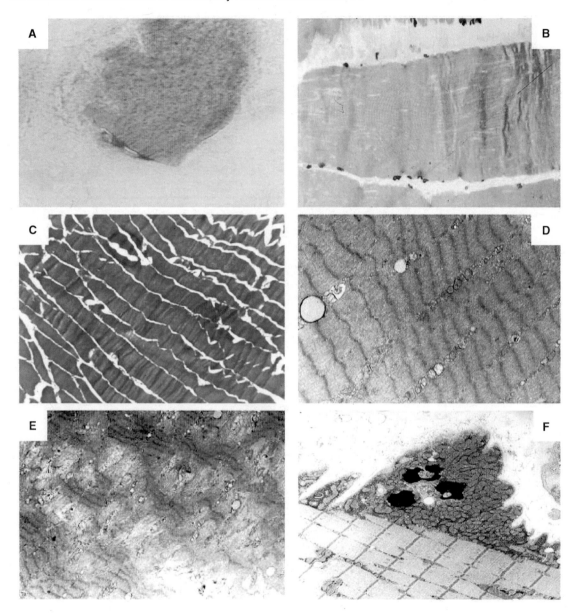

REFERENCES

1. Engel, AG, Franzini-Armstrong C: Myology. Second Edition, Vol 1. and 2. McGraw-Hill, Inc., New York, USA, 1994.

2. Karpati, G: Structural and molecular basis of skeletal muscle diseases. ISN Neuropath Press, Basel, Swiss, 2002.

3. Karpati, G, Hilton-Jones, D, Griggs RG: Disorders of voluntary muscle. Oxford University Press, New York, USA, 2001.

4. Figarella-Branger D, Civatte M, Bartoli C, Pellissier JF: Cytokines, chemokines, and cell adhesion molecules in inflammatory myopathies. Muscle & Nerve 28: 659-682, 2003.

5. Dalakas MC, Hohlfeld R: Polymyositis and dermatomyositis. Lancet 362: 1762-1763, 2003.

6. Askanas V, Engel WK: Proposed pathogenetic cascade of inclusion-body myositis: Importance of amyloid-beta, misfold proteins, predisposing gene, and aging. Curr Opin Rheumatol 15: 737-744, 2003.

7. Argov, Z, Lofberg M, Arnold DL: Insights into muscle diseases gained by phosphorus magnetic resonance spectroscopy. Muscle & Nerve 23: 1316-1333, 2002.

8. Wolfsdorf JI, Weinstein DA: Glycogen storage diseases. Rev Endocr Metab Disord 4: 95-102, 2003.

9. Vorgerd M, Zange J: Carbohydrate oxidation disorders of skeletal muscle. Curr Opin Clin Nutr Metab Care 5:611-617, 2002.

10. Norman B, Mahnke-Zizelman DK, Vallis A, Sabina RL: Genetic and other determinants of AMP deaminase activity in healthy adult skeletal muscle. J Appl Physiol 85: 1273-1278, 1998.

11. Sabina RL: Myoadenylate deaminase deficiency. A common inherited defect with heterogeneous clinical presentation. Neurol Clin 18: 185-194, 2000.

12. Gerwin RD: Classification, epidemiology, and natural history of myofascial pain syndrome. Curr Pain Headache Rep. 5: 412-420, 2001.

13. Simons DG: Review of enigmatic MTrPs as a common cause of enigmatic musculoskeletal pain and dysfunction. J Electromyogr Kinesiol. 14: 95-107, 2004.

14. Reilich, P, Pongratz, D: Myofascial pain syndrome. In: Jost WH (ed.): Botulinum toxin in painful diseases, pain headache. Karger, Basel, Swiss, pp. 23-41, 2003.

Index

Acetylcholine release, TrPs due to, 16
Acid maltase deficiency, 80
ACR. *See* American College of Rheumatology (ACR)
ACTH. *See* Adrenocorticotrophin (ACTH)
Acupuncture
    in fibromyalgia management, 67
    for myofascial pain, 41
Adrenocorticotrophin (ACTH), for FMS, 5
Allergy(ies), myalgia due to, 26
Alternative therapy, for idiopathic LBP, 116
American College of Rheumatology (ACR), 49
American College of Rheumatology (ACR) research
    classification criteria, for fibromyalgia
    syndrome, 59-62. *See also* Fibromyalgia
    syndrome (FMS), ACR research
    classification criteria for
Antibody(ies), antipolymer, in pathogenesis of
    fibromyalgia syndrome, 51-52
Anti-Mi-2, features of, 86t
Antipolymer antibodies, in pathogenesis of
    fibromyalgia syndrome, 51-52
Anti-SRP, features of, 86t
Anti-synthetases, features of, 86t
Autoimmune disorders, myalgia due to, 25
Autonomic dysfunction, in FMS, 5-6
Azathioprine, for IIMs, 89

Back pain, low, idiopathic, 93-99. *See also* Low back
    pain (LBP), idiopathic
Balneotherapy, in fibromyalgia management, 68
Bartels, E.M., 93
Bauermeister, W., 15,18,19,19t
Bed rest, for idiopathic LBP, 113
Bennett, R.M., 1,59
Biofeedback, in fibromyalgia management, 68
Biological markers, in pathogenesis of fibromyalgia
    syndrome, 51-52
Blackman, J.G., 17
Bliddal, H., 111
Botulinum toxin (BTX) injections
    for myofascial pain, 7
    for TrPs, 41
Brain tumor, base of skull pain due to, 26
Brody's disease, 81
Bruxism, MMP and, 31
BTX injections. *See* Botulinum toxin (BTX) injections
Burckhardt, C.S., 65

CAM. *See* Complementary and alternative medicine
    (CAM)
Cancer-associated myositis, features of, 86t
Cathechol-*O*-methyltransferase (COMT), FMS and,
    6-7
CBT. *See* Cognitive-behavioral therapy (CBT)
Cell(s), glial, in central sensitization induced by
    painful muscle lesion, 106-108,107f
Central nervous system (CNS), local muscle pain
    effects on, 101-109
Central sensitization
    in FMS, 3-4,3t
    neurotransmitters involved in, 103
    painful muscle lesions and, glial cells in,
    106-108,107f
CFS. *See* Chronic fatigue syndrome (CFS)
Chronic fatigue syndrome (CFS), 49
Chronic progressive external ophthalmoplegia, 81
Clinical Center of the National Institutes of Health,
    Department of Rehabilitation Medicine of, 18
CNS. *See* Central nervous system (CNS)
Cognitive-behavioral therapy (CAT)
    for chronic myalgia, 34
    in fibromyalgia management, 66
Cold application, for myofascial pain, 40
COMP. *See* Cathechol-*O*-methyltransferase (COMT)
Complementary and alternative medicine (CAM), for
    fibromyalgia, 65-66
Connective tissue myositis, features of, 86t
Contracture(s), in metabolic myopathies, 79
Corticosteroid(s), for IIMs, 89
Corticotropin releasing hormone (CRH), for FMS, 5
Cramp(s), muscle, in metabolic myopathies, 79
CRH. *See* Corticotropin releasing hormone (CRH)
Crofford, L., 73
Cytokine(s)
    in FMS, 4-5
    in pathogenesis of fibromyalgia syndrome, 51-52
    in stress disorders, 2

Danneskiold-Samsoe, B., 93
Daubert v. Merrell Dow, 56
    delete 219, myofascial trigger point(s) (TrP(s))
    clinical developments in, 18-20,18t,19t
    clusters of, 19-20
    identification of
        diagnostic examinations in, 19

interrater reliability of examiners for, 19
 shockwave devices for, 18-19,19t
increased fiber tension and, 17,17t
injection for, 40-41
interactions of, 19-20
introduction to, 15
loci of, 37-38
new aspects of, 15-21
pathophysiological features of, 16,16f
sensitizing substances and, 17
tissue milieu of, study of, 18,18t
Department of Rehabilitation Medicine, of Clinical
 Center of the National Institutes of Health, 18
"De-Qui" effect, 41
Dermatomyositis
 clinical signs of, 122,123f
 features of, 86t
Diet(s), in fibromyalgia management, 68-69
Dietary supplements, in fibromyalgia management,
 68-69
Disaster(s), World Trade Center, psychological
 distress due to, 1-2
Drug(s)
 for chronic myalgia, 34
 for fibromyalgia syndrome, 54-55
 for idiopathic LBP, 115-116
 for MMP, 33
 myalgia due to, 27
Dry needling, for myofascial pain, 41
Duloxetine, for fibromyalgia syndrome, 55

Education, patient, in fibromyalgia management, 66
Ehlers-Danlos syndrome, 24
ELAS. *See* Mitochondrial myopathy, encephalopathy,
 lactate acidosis, and stroke-like episodes
 (MELAS)
Electrical muscle stimulation, for myofascial pain, 40
Electrical nerve stimulation, for myofascial pain, 40
Energy metabolism, in muscle, 76-78,77f
Enzyme(s), respiratory chain, defects of, 81
Exercise(s)
 extension, for idiopathic LBP, 113-114
 in fibromyalgia management, 66-67
 myalgia due to, 24,80
Extension exercises, for idiopathic LBP, 113-114

Fatigue, in FMS, 5
Fiber tension, increased, TrPs due to, 17,17t
Fibromyalgia Impact Questionnaire (FIQ), 3
Fibromyalgia Impact Questionnaire (FIQ) total score,
 67
Fibromyalgia syndrome (FMS), 1
 ACR research classification criteria for, 59-62
  classification in, 61
  problems with, 61-62

revised criteria, 62
 study design, 60
 study results, 60-61
Canadian clinical case definition of, 49-50
central sensitization in, 3-4,3t
COMP and, 6-7
cytokines in, 4-5
death due to, 56
described, 3,47
developments in, 47-57
diagnosis of, 48-50,48t,49f,59-62. *See also*
 Fibromyalgia syndrome (FMS), ACR
 research classification criteria for
differential diagnosis of, 62-63,63t
epidemiological studies of, 2-3
errant terminology in, 48
fatigue in, 5
genetic studies of, 6-7
legal issues related to, 56
management of, 54-56
 ACTH in, 5
 acupuncture in, 67
 balneotherapy in, 68
 biofeedback in, 68
 CAM in, 65-66
 CBT in, 66
 CRH in, 5
 diet in, 68-69
 dietary supplement in, 68-69
 drugs in, 54-55
  novel agents, 73
 duloxetine in, 55
 evaluation of, 69-70
 exercise in, 66-67
 HGH in, 55
 magnets, 69
 metyrapone in, 5
 milnacipran in, 55
 movement therapies in, 68
 multicomponent strategies in, 67
 novel approaches to, 65-72
 patient education in, 66
 pregabalin in, 55
 pyridostigmine in, 5-6,55
 RCTs in, 66
 recommendations for, 69-70
 SEA in, 7
 surgical, 55-56
natural history of, 56
neuroendocrine and autonomic dysfunction in, 5-6
9/11 and, 2
1990 American College of Rheumatology
 classification criteria for, 59-62
overlap, *vs.* subgroups, 50-51,50f
pathogenesis of, 50-54,50f
 antipolymer antibodies in, 51-52
 biological markers in, 51-52

cytokines in, 51-52
genetic issues in, 52-53
GPCRs in, 53-54,53f
pure as possible for, 51
subgroups, *vs.* overlap, 50-51,50f
tizanidine in, 54
psychological stressors and, 1
research classification of, 49
soft tissue pain classification in, 48-49,48t,49f
trigger points in, 7
FIQ. *See* Fibromyalgia Impact Questionnaire (FIQ)
FMS. *See* Fibromoyalgia syndrome (FMS)
Forward head posture, myalgia due to, 24

G protein–coupled receptors (GPCRs), in fibromyalgia
syndrome, 53-54,53f
Genetic issues, in fibromyalgia syndrome, 52-53
Genetic studies, in FMS, 6-7
Gerwin, R., 23
Glial cells, in central sensitization induced by painful
muscle lesion, 106-108,107f
Glycogenolysis, defects of, 80
Glycogenosis type V, clinical signs of, 125,126f
Glycolysis, defects of, 80
GPCRs. *See* G protein–coupled receptors (GPCRs)

Head posture, forward, myalgia due to, 24
Health Canada, 49-50
HGH. *See* Human growth hormone (HGH)
Hoheisel, U., 101
Hong, C-Z, 37
Human growth hormone (HGH), for fibromyalgia
syndrome, 55
Hypermobility syndromes, 24

Idiopathic inflammatory myopathies (IIMs), 85-91
clinical presentation of, 86-87,87t
introduction to, 85-86,86f
poor prognostic factors in, 87,88t
treatment of, 87-90,88t-90t
assessment of disease activity and damage in, 88
azathioprine in, 89
corticosteroids in, 89
general considerations in, 87-88,88t
methotrexate in, 89
physical therapy in, 90
rehabilitation in, 90
Idiopathic LBP, 93-99. *See also* Low back pain (LBP),
idiopathic
treatment of, 111-119. *See also* Low back pain
(LBP), idiopathic, treatment of
Idiopathic polymyositis, clinical signs of, 122,124f
IIMs. *See* Idiopathic inflammatory myopathies (IIMs)
IMACS. *See* International Myositis Assessment and
Clinical Studies Group (IMACS)

IMS. *See* International MYOPAIN Society (IMS)
Incidence, defined, 94
Inclusion body myositis, features of, 86t
Infectious diseases, myalgia due to, 26
Inherited metabolic myopathies, clinical signs of,
125,126f
International MYOPAIN Society (IMS), 1
Sixth World Congress of, xiii
International Myositis Assessment and Clinical Studies
Group (IMACS), 88
Intramuscular stimulation, for myofascial pain, 41
Iron deficiency, TrPs and, 27

JNKs. *See* c-Jun N-terminal kinases (JNKs)
Journal of Musculoskeletal Pain, 1
c-Jun N-terminal kinases (JNKs), 5
Juvenile myositis, features of, 86t

Laser therapy, for myofascial pain, 40
LBP. *See* Low back pain (LBP)
Legal issues, fibromyalgia syndrome–related, 56
Lewit, K., 19
Life-time prevalence, defined, 94
Lipid metabolism, defects of, 81
Local myosfascial pain syndrome, clinical signs of,
125,127f
London Fibromyalgia Epidemiology Study Group, 2,3
Low back pain (LBP)
clinical course of, 95
defined, 93
described, 93-94
diagnosis of, 95-97,97f
differential diagnosis of, 95-97,97f
epidemiologic features of, 94-95
genetic influences of, 94-95
idiopathic, 93-99
introduction to, 111-112,112f
recurrence of, prevention of, 115
risk factors for, 95
treatment of, 111-119
alternative therapy, 116
bed rest, 113
extension exercises, 113-114
manipulation, 115
pharmacologic, 115-116
selection criteria, 116-117
surgery, 116
types of, 112-113
imaging of, 96
incidence of, 94-95
introduction to, 93-94
non-specific, classification of, 96-97,97f
pain with, 97
pathological features of, 95
possible confounders in, 112

prevalence of, 95
    regional pain disorders in, 113,114t
Lyme disease, myalgia due to, 26

MADA. *See* Myoadenylate deaminase (MADA)
Magnet(s), in fibromyalgia management, 69
Manipulation, for idiopathic LBP, 115
MAPK. *See* Mitogen-activated protein kinase (MAPK)
Martinez-Lavin, M., 6
Massage, therapeutic, in fibromyalgia management, 68
Masticatory myofascial pain (MMP)
    bruxism and, 31
    cause of, 30
    diagnosis of, 31-32
    episodic, 30
    non-chronic form of, treatment of, 32-34,33f
    treatment of, 32-34,33f
        occlusal appliances in, 33-34,33f
        pharmacologic, 33
        physiotherapy in, 33
        relaxation therapy in, 33
        trigger point needling in, 34
    TrPs and, 30-31
McArdle disease, 80
    clinical signs of, 125,126f
"Memory traces," of pain, 13
Mense, S., 17,101
MERRF syndrome, 8
Metabolic myopathies
    inherited, clinical signs of, 125,126f
    myalgias due to, treatment of, 82
Metabolic myopathyies, muscle pain in, pathogenesis
        of, 78,79f. *See also* Muscle pain, in
        metabolic myopathies
Methotrexate, for IIMs, 89
Metyrapone, for FMS, 5
Miller, F.W., 85
Milnacipran, for fibromyalgia syndrome, 55
Mitochondrial myopathy, encephalopathy, lactate
        acidosis, and stroke-like episodes (MELAS),
        81
Mitogen-activated protein kinase (MAPK), 5
MMP. *See* Masticatory myofascial pain (MMP)
Movement therapies, in fibromyalgia management, 68
MPDS. *See* Myofascial pain dysfunction syndromes
        (MPDS)
Muscle(s), energy metabolism in, 76-78,77f
Muscle disorders, 80-81
    acid maltase deficiency, 80
    Brody's disease, 81
    chronic progressive external ophthalmoplegia, 81
    glycogenolysis defects, 80
    glycolysis defects, 80
    lipid metabolism defects
    MADA deficiency, 81
    McArdle syndrome, 80

MELAS, 81
    MERRF syndrome, 81
    phosphofructokinase defects, 80
    respiratory chain enzyme defects, 81
    Tarui disease, 80
Muscle imbalance, myalgia due to, 25
Muscle lesion(s), painful, central sensitization induced
        by, glial cells in, 106-108,107f
Muscle pain. *See also specific disorders*
    chronic, NO–CGMP axis as factor in,
        103-106,104f-106f
    clinical signs of, 121-128
    local, CNS sequelae of, 101-109
    in metabolic myopathies
        contractures, 79
        cramps, 79
        myotonia, 79-80
        pathogenesis of, 78,79f
        specific diseases, 80-81. *See also specific
            disorders*
        types of, 79-80
    scientific aspects of, 121-128
Muscle Pain, 17
Myalgia(s)
    causes of, 23-25,75,76,76t
        allergies, 26
        autoimmune disorders, 25
        base of skull pain, 26
        brain tumor, 26
        exercise, 24
        hypermobility syndromes, 24
        infectious diseases, 26
        Lyme disease, 26
        medical, 25
        muscle imbalance, 25
        nerve root compression, 25
        pelvic torsion–related, 24
        sacroiliac joint dysfunction, 24-25
        somatic dysfunction, 25
        static overload, 25
        viscero-somatic pain syndromes, 26
    characteristics of, 76
    chronic, management of, 34
    classification of, 75-76,76t
    defined, 23
    drug-induced, 27
    exercise-induced, 80
    metabolic myopathies and, treatment of, 82
    pathogenesis of, 75
    prevalence of, 75
    TrPs and, 23-26
Myoadenylate deaminase (MADA), deficiency of, 81
Myoclonic encephalopathy with ragged-red-fibers
        (MERRF) syndrome, 81
Myofascial pain, 7
    BTX injections for, 7
    described, 29

masticatory, TrPs and, 30-31
treatment of, 37-43
    acupuncture in, 41
    basic principle of, 38-40,39t
    mechanism of, 38
    physical therapy in, 40
underlying pathological lesions in, identification
    and treatment of, 38
Myofascial pain dysfunction syndromes (MPDS), 48
Myofascial pain syndrome, features of, 23
Myofascial trigger point(s) (TrP(s))
    acetylcholine release and, 16
    active, inactivation of, 39-40,39t
    causes of, 16-17,16f,17t
Myofascial trigger point (TrP) injection, 40-41
    Fischer's technique of, 41
    general principles of, 40-41
MYOPAIN 2004, xiii,1-12
    peripheral pain generators in, 4
Myopathy(ies)
    idiopathic inflammatory, 85-91. *See also* Idiopathic
        inflammatory myopathies (IIMs)
    metabolic. *See* Metabolic myopathies
    painful, 75-119. *See also specific disorder*
Myositis
    cancer-associated, features of, 86t
    connective tissue, features of, 86t
    inclusion body, features of, 86t
    juvenile, features of, 86t
    neuroplastic changes in spinal dorsal horn due to,
        102-103,102f
    sporadic inclusion body, clinical signs of, 122,124f
Myotonia, in metabolic myopathies, 79-80

National Institutes of Health (NIH), 15
Neeck, G., 45
Nerve root compression, myalgia due to, 25
Neue Pinakothek Museum of Fine Art, xiii
Neuroendocrine dysfunction, in FMS, 5-6
Neuroendocrine system, pain and, 45
Neurotransmitter(s), in central sensitization, 103
NIH. *See* National Institutes of Health (NIH)
9/11. *See* September 11, 2001
Nitric oxide–cyclic guanosine monophosphate
        (NO–CGMP) axis, as factor in chronic
        muscle pain, 103-106,104f-106f
NO–CGMP axis. *See* Nitric oxide–cyclic guanosine
        monophosphate (NO–CGMP) axis
Nutritional deficiencies
    iron deficiency, 27
    TrPs and, 26-27
    vitamin D deficiency, 26

Occlusal appliances, for MMP, 33-34,33f
Ophthalmoplegia, chronic progressive external, 81

Orofacial pain
    described, 29
    prevalence of, 29
    TrPs and, 29-36
        treatment of, 32-34,33f

Pain
    from acute to chronic
        mechanisms of, 13
        transition from, 106
    back, low, idiopathic, 93-99. See also Low back
        pain (LBP), idiopathic
    base of skull, brain tumor and, 26
    "memory traces" of, 13
    muscle. *See* Muscle pain
        local, CNS sequelae of, 101-109
    myofascial. *See* Myofascial pain
    neuroendocrine system and, 45
    orofacial, TrPs and, 29-36
    pelvic torsion–related, myalgia due to, 24
Pain disorders, regional, in LBP, 113,114t
Pain referral, types of, 30
Painful muscle lesions, central sensitization induced
        by, glial cells in, 106-108,107f
Palla, S., 29
Patient education, in fibromyalgia management, 66
Pelvic torsion–related pain, myalgia due to, 24
Period prevalence, defined, 94
Peripheral pain generators, 4
Phosphofructokinase, defects in, 80
Phosphorylase deficiency, clinical signs of, 125,126f
Physical therapy
    for IIMs, 90
    for myofascial pain, 40
Physiotherapy, for MMP, 33
Point prevalence, defined, 94
Polymyositis
    features of, 86t
    idiopathic, clinical signs of, 122,124f
Pongratz, D.E., 121
Post-traumatic stress disorder (PTSD), war and, 1
Posture, head, forward, myalgia due to, 24
Pregabalin, for fibromyalgia syndrome, 55
Prevalence
    life-time, defined, 94
    period, defined, 94
    point, defined, 94
Psychological distress, WTC disaster and, 1-2
Psychological stressors, FMS due to, 1-2
PTSD. *See* Post-traumatic stress disorder (PTSD)
Pyridostigmine, for FMS, 5-6,55

Randomized controlled trials (RCTs), in fibromyalgia
        management, 66
RCTs. *See* Randomized controlled trials (RCTs)

Regional pain disorders, in LBP, 113,114t
Regionalized syndromes, 48
Rehabilitation, for IIMs, 90
Reichmann, H., 75
Relaxation therapy, for MMP, 33
Respiratory chain enzymes, defects of, 81
Russell, I.J., xiii,47

Sacroiliac joint dysfunction, myalgia due to, 24-25
Schaefer, J., 75
Schoser, B.G.H., 121
SEA. *See* Spontaneous electrical activity (SEA)
Selye, 2
Sensitization, central. *See* Central sensitization
Sensitizing substances, TrPs due to, 17
September 11, 2001, FMS due to, 2
Shah, J., 15,18
Shockwave devices, TrPs-related, 18-19,19t
Simons, D.G., 15,17
Skull, base of, pain of, brain tumor and, 26
Soft tissue pain (STP) syndromes, classification of,
     48-49,48t,49f
Somatic dysfunction, myalgia due to, 25
Spinal dorsal horn, myositis-induced neuroplastic
     changes in, 102-103,102f
Spontaneous electrical activity (SEA), for FMS, 7
Sporadic inclusion body myositis, clinical signs of,
     122,124f
Static overload, myalgia due to, 25
Stolov, W.C., 17
Stress disorders, cytokines in, 2
Stressor(s), psychological, FMS due to, 1-2

Tarui disease, 80
Tender points, TrPs *vs.*, 29
"The-Chi" effect, 41
Therapeutic massage, in fibromyalgia management, 68
Thermotherapy, for myofascial pain, 40
Tizanidine, for FMS, 54
Trigger point needling, for MMP, 34
Trigger points (TrPs)
     clinical characteristics of, 29-30
     differential diagnosis of, 23-28
     in FMS, 7
     myalgia and, 23-26
     myofascial. *See* Myofascial trigger points (TrPs)
     nutritional deficiencies and, 26-27
     orofacial pain due to, 29-36
     tender points *vs.*, 29
TrP injection, 40-41
TrPs. *See* Myofascial trigger points (TrPs); Trigger
     points (TrPs)
Tumor(s), brain, base of skull pain due to, 26

Viscero-soamtic pain syndromes, myalgia due to, 26
Vitamin D deficiency, TrPs and, 26
Vorgerd, M., 121

War, PTSD due to, 1
"Widespread pain" (WSP), 49
World Trade Center disaster, psychological distress
     due to, 1-2
WSP. *See* "Widespread pain" (WSP)

Zieglgänsberger, W., 13

BOOK ORDER FORM!

Order a copy of this book with this form or online at:
http://www.haworthpress.com/store/product.asp?sku=5764

Soft Tissue Pain Syndromes
Clinical Diagnosis and Pathogenesis

____ in softbound at $24.95 ISBN-13: 978-0-7890-3138-9 / ISBN-10: 0-7890-3138-8.

COST OF BOOKS _____

POSTAGE & HANDLING _____
US: $4.00 for first book & $1.50
for each additional book
Outside US: $5.00 for first book
& $2.00 for each additional book.

SUBTOTAL _____

In Canada: add 7% GST. _____

STATE TAX _____
CA, IL, IN, MN, NJ, NY, OH, PA & SD residents
please add appropriate local sales tax.

FINAL TOTAL _____
If paying in Canadian funds, convert
using the current exchange rate,
UNESCO coupons welcome.

❑**BILL ME LATER:**
Bill-me option is good on US/Canada/
Mexico orders only; not good to jobbers,
wholesalers, or subscription agencies.

❑**Signature** _____

❑ **Payment Enclosed: $** _____

❑ **PLEASE CHARGE TO MY CREDIT CARD:**

❑Visa ❑MasterCard ❑AmEx ❑Discover
❑Diner's Club ❑Eurocard ❑ JCB

Account #_____

Exp Date _____

Signature _____
(Prices in US dollars and subject to change without notice.)

PLEASE PRINT ALL INFORMATION OR ATTACH YOUR BUSINESS CARD
Name
Address
City   State/Province   Zip/Postal Code
Country
Tel   Fax
E-Mail

May we use your e-mail address for confirmations and other types of information? ❑Yes ❑No We appreciate receiving
your e-mail address. Haworth would like to e-mail special discount offers to you, as a preferred customer.
We will never share, rent, or exchange your e-mail address. We regard such actions as an invasion of your privacy.

Order from your **local bookstore** or directly from
The Haworth Press, Inc. 10 Alice Street, Binghamton, New York 13904-1580 • USA
Call our toll-free number (1-800-429-6784) / Outside US/Canada: (607) 722-5857
Fax: 1-800-895-0582 / Outside US/Canada: (607) 771-0012
E-mail your order to us: orders@haworthpress.com

For orders outside US and Canada, you may wish to order through your local
sales representative, distributor, or bookseller.
For information, see http://haworthpress.com/distributors

(Discounts are available for individual orders in US and Canada only, not booksellers/distributors.)

The Haworth Press Inc.

Please photocopy this form for your personal use.
www.HaworthPress.com

BOF05